Graduate Education in Internal Medicine

A Resource Guide to Curriculum Development

D1372452

The Report of the
FEDERATED COUNCIL FOR
INTERNAL MEDICINE TASK FORCE
ON THE INTERNAL MEDICINE RESIDENCY CURRICULUM

Graduate Education in Internal Medicine

A Resource Guide to Curriculum Development

The Report of the
FEDERATED COUNCIL FOR
INTERNAL MEDICINE TASK FORCE
ON THE INTERNAL MEDICINE RESIDENCY CURRICULUM

EDITORS

Jack Ende, MD
The University of Pennsylvania

Mark A. Kelley, MD
The University of Pennsylvania

Paul G. Ramsey, MD
The University of Washington

Harold C. Sox, MD (Task Force Chair)
Dartmouth Medical School

CONTRIBUTING EDITORS

Francois M. Abboud, MD
The University of Iowa

Richard D. Ruppert, MD
Medical College of Ohio

Beverly Woo, MD
Harvard Medical School

Robert E. Wright, MD
Scranton-Temple Residency Program

MANAGER, BOOKS PROGRAM: David Myers
COVER DESIGNER: Michael Ripca
TEXT DESIGNER: Patricia Wieland

Printed in the United States of America.

COMPOSITION by Patricia Wieland
PRINTING by Versa Press

Library of Congress Cataloging-in-Publication Data

Graduate education in internal medicine : a resource guide to curriculum
    development / report of the Federated Council for Internal Medicine,
    Task Force on the Internal Medicine Residency Curriculum : editors,
    Harold Sox . . . [et al.].
        p.   cm.
    Cover title.
    ISBN 0-943126-60-6 (alk. paper)
    1. Internal medicine—Study and teaching (Residency)—Handbooks,
manuals, etc. 2. Medical education—Philosophy—Handbooks, manuals,
etc. I. Sox, Harold C. II. Federated Council for Internal
Medicine. Task Force on the Internal Medicine Residency Curriculum.
    [DNLM: 1. Internal Medicine—education. 2. Education, Medical,
Graduate. 3. Curriculum. WB 18 G733 1997]
RC737.G66   1997
616'.0071'55—dc21
DNLM/DLC
for Library of Congress   97-3199
                                                        CIP

To order copies of *Graduate Education in Internal Medicine*, contact:

Customer Service Center
American College of Physicians
Independence Mall West
Sixth Street at Race
Philadelphia, PA 19106-1572
215-351-2600
800-523-1546, ext. 2600

5 4 3 2 1

CONTENTS

ACKNOWLEDGMENTS

Many individuals helped the Task Force in its work. You will see here the names of practicing internists and department of medicine chairs, residency program directors and teachers, subspecialists and general internists, rural internists and urban internists, experienced practitioners and newly minted internists. Some of these individuals wrote draft competency lists, which the editors combined into a single list. Others participated in a systematic review organized by the Task Force to include the perspectives of residency program directors, subspecialists, and general internists newly in practice. Still others reviewed the competency lists for their subspecialty society or simply wrote to us after reading a stray copy of early drafts of the report. Some people made important conceptual contributions to the project. Rather than single out any person for special recognition, we list everyone that our records list as having contributed. Omissions are inevitable in such a large undertaking. We will correct them in subsequent printings.

The American College of Physicians Education Division provided the staff support for this project. We owe special thanks to Susan Deutsch, MD, and Glynis Rhodes, who, respectively, directed and provided the logistical support for the project. David Smines, Dalia Ritter, and Peter Dorman prepared and edited the manuscript. Herbert Waxman, MD, and Frank Davidoff, MD, Theresa Kanya, and Kathy Egan, PhD, provided steadfast overall direction for the Education Division during the project. We received help from the Clerkship Directors in Internal Medicine through the counsel of Gail Morrison, MD.

The Task Force could not have completed its task without financial support from the organizations that compose the Federated Council for Internal Medicine and grants from the Robert Wood Johnson Foundation and the Josiah Macy Foundation.

Thanks to all for participating in a grand collaboration of the greatest significance for our discipline. You have helped to define the internist. Your colleagues everywhere will hold you in high esteem for your contribution.

Members of the Task Force:

Francois M. Abboud, MD, for the Association of Professors of Medicine

Jack Ende, MD, for the Association of Program Directors in Internal Medicine

Mark A. Kelley, MD, for the American Board of Internal Medicine

Paul G. Ramsey, MD, for the Association of Professors of Medicine

Richard D. Ruppert, MD, for the American Society of Internal Medicine

Harold C. Sox, MD (Chair), for the American College of Physicians

Beverly Woo, MD, for the Society for General Internal Medicine

Robert E. Wright, MD, for the Association of Program Directors in Internal Medicine

N. Franklin Adkinson, Jr., MD
Johns Hopkins University School of
    Medicine
Baltimore, Maryland

Joseph S. Alpert, MD
University of Arizona School of Medicine
Tucson, Arizona

Ernest N. Arnett, MD
Franklin Square Hospital Center
Baltimore, Maryland

Robert M. Arnold, MD
University of Pittsburgh
Pittsburgh, Pennsylvania

Gerard P. Aurigemma, MD
University of Massachusetts Medical
    Center
Worcester, Massachusetts

David Babbott, MD
Burlington, Vermont

Erin L. Bakanas, MD
St. Louis University
St. Louis, Missouri

Mark Ballow, MD
Children's Hospital of Buffalo
Buffalo, New York

Thomas W. Barber, MD
Boston City Hospital
Boston, Massachusetts

Emil J. Bardana, Jr., MD
Oregon Health Sciences University
Portland, Oregon

William Barron, MD
Loyola University Medical Center
Maywood, Illinois

Patricia P. Barry, MD, MPH
Boston University Medical Center
    Hospital
Boston, Massachusetts

John G. Bartlett, MD
Johns Hopkins Hospital
Baltimore, Maryland

Christine Bastl, MD
National Kidney Foundation
New York, New York

Paul Batalden, MD
Dartmouth-Hitchcock Medical Center
Lebanon, New Hampshire

David Battinelli, MD
University Hospital
Boston, Massachusetts

William G. Baxt, MD
Hospital of the University of Pennsylvania
Philadelphia, Pennsylvania

John C. Beck, MD
University of California, Los Angeles
Los Angeles, California

J. Claude Bennett, MD
BioCryst Pharmaceuticals
Birmingham, Alabama

Lee R. Berkowitz, MD
University of North Carolina
Chapel Hill, North Carolina

Donald Berwick, MD
Newton, Massachusetts

Linda Blank
American Board of Internal Medicine
Philadelphia, Pennsylvania

Joseph R. Bloomer, MD
University of Alabama at Birmingham
Birmingham, Alabama

John Wolfe Blotzer, MD
York Hospital
York, Pennsylvania

Leslie F. Blum, MD
Norwalk Hospital
Norwalk, Connecticut

Maj. Charles Bolan, MD
Walter Reed Army Medical Center
Washington, D.C.

Peter Boling, MD
Medical College of Virginia
Richmond, Virginia

Judith Bowen, MD
Virginia Mason Medical Center
Seattle, Washington

Richard D. Brasington, Jr., MD
Washington University School of
    Medicine
St. Louis, Missouri

Martin I. Broder, MD
Baystate Medical Center
Springfield, Massachusetts

Michael Bronze, MD
University of Tennessee
Memphis, Tennessee

Patricia Brown, MD
Detroit Medical Center
Detroit, Michigan

Helen Burstin, MD
Brigham and Women's Hospital
Boston, Massachusetts

Richard Campbell, MD
Methodist Hospital of Indiana
Indianapolis, Indiana

Thomas W. Cann III, MD
York, Pennsylvania

Joan I. Casey, MD
Montefiore Hospital and Medical Center
New York, New York

Christine Cassel, MD
Mt. Sinai Medical Center
New York, New York

Peter Cassileth, MD
University of Miami School of Medicine
Miami, Florida

Jean A. Chapman, MD
Cape Girardeau, Missouri

Pamela Charney, MD
Albert Einstein College of Medicine
Bronx, New York

Melvin D. Cheitlin, MD
San Francisco General Hospital
San Francisco, California

Lawrence T. Chiaramonte, MD
Long Island College of Medicine
Little Neck, New York

Richard E. Christie, MD
St. Luke's Medical Center
Cleveland, Ohio

Joseph P. Cleary, MD
Norwalk Hospital
Norwalk, Connecticut

David M. Clive, MD
University of Massachusetts
Worcester, Massachusetts

M. S. Cohen, MD

Steven Cole, MD
Long Island Jewish Medical Center
Glen Oaks, New York

Barry S. Coller, MD
Mt. Sinai Medical Center
New York, New York

Virginia U. Collier, MD
Medical Center of Delaware
Newark, Delaware

Victor A. Collymore, MD
Englewood, Colorado

Erik Constance, MD
Springfield, Illinois

Thomas G. Cooney, MD
Oregon Health Sciences University
Portland, Oregon

Anthony M. Cosentino, MD
St. Mary's Medical Center
San Francisco, California

Steven R. Counsell, MD
SUMMA Health System
Akron, Ohio

David R. Dantzker, MD
Long Island Jewish Medical Center
New Hyde Park, New York

Peter Davidson, MD
Washington University School of
   Medicine
St. Louis, Missouri

Faith B. Davis, MD
Albany Medical College
Albany, New York

Paul J. Davis, MD
Albany Medical College
Albany, New York

Vincent A. DeLuca, MD
Griffin Hospital
Derby, Connecticut

Michele E. DeMusis, MD
Greater Baltimore Medical Center
Baltimore, Maryland

Richard deShazo, MD
University of South Alabama
Mobile, Alabama

Herbert S. Diamond, MD
Western Pennsylvania Hospital
Pittsburgh, Pennsylvania

William Dismukes, MD
University of Alabama at Birmingham
Birmingham, Alabama

Glenda D. Donoghue, MD
Medical College of Pennsylvania and
   Hahnemann
Philadelphia, Pennsylvania

Janice Douglas, MD
Case Western Reserve University
Cleveland, Ohio

Jack R. Ebright, MD
Wayne State University
Detroit, Michigan

Thomas E. Edes, MD
Harry S. Truman Memorial Veterans
   Affairs Hospital
Columbia, Missouri

Adrian Edwards, MD
New York Hospital
New York, New York

Joseph Eron, MD

Emily Fairchild, MD
University of Maryland School of
   Medicine
Baltimore, Maryland

Robert P. Ferguson, MD
Union Memorial Hospital
Baltimore, Maryland

Tom Finucane, MD
Johns Hopkins University School of
   Medicine
Baltimore, Maryland

Rosemarie L. Fisher, MD
Yale–New Haven Medical Center
New Haven, Connecticut

Robert H. Fletcher, MD
Harvard Medical School
Boston, Massachusetts

Eric M. Flint, MD
Mt. Auburn Hospital
Cambridge, Massachusetts

Robert Forman, MD
Albert Einstein College of Medicine
New York, New York

Ellen Fox, MD
University of Illinois at Chicago
Chicago, Illinois

Charles K. Francis, MD
Harlem Hospital Center
New York, New York

Harold M. Friedman, MD
Dartmouth-Hitchcock Medical Center
Lebanon, New Hampshire

Lawrence Friedman, MD
Massachusetts General Hospital
Boston, Massachusetts

Robert Frye, MD
Mayo Medical School
Rochester, Minnesota

Morton Fuchs, MD
Tucson Hospitals and Medical Education
Tucson, Arizona

Timothy F. Gabryel, MD
Millard Fillmore Hospital
Buffalo, New York

Nancy Gagliano, MD
Massachusetts General Hospital
Boston, Massachusetts

William B. Galbraith, MD
University of Iowa Hospitals and Clinics
Iowa City, Iowa

Susan J. Gallagher, MD
Amherst, New York

Richard A. Garabaldi, MD
University of Connecticut
Farmington, Connecticut

Raymond A. Gensinger, Jr., MD
Minneapolis, Minnesota

Andrew S. Gersoff, MD
Santa Barbara Cottage Hospital
Santa Barbara, California

William Golden, MD
University of Arkansas School of Medicine
Little Rock, Arkansas

David R. Goldmann, MD
American College of Physicians
Philadelphia, Pennsylvania

Harvey M. Golomb, MD
University of Chicago Medical Center
Chicago, Illinois

Sarah J. Goodlin, MD
Veterans Affairs Hospital
White River Junction, Vermont

Roseanne Gramier, MD
University of Pittsburgh
Pittsburgh, Pennsylvania

Gary Green, MD
UCLA Center for the Health Sciences
Los Angeles, California

Michael Green, MD
Hershey Medical Center
Hershey, Pennsylvania

Michael J. Greene, MD
University of Wisconsin
Hummelstown, Pennsylvania

Ruth Hanft, PhD
Alexandria, Virginia

Daniel C. Hardesty, MD
Franklin Square Hospital Center
Baltimore, Maryland

Charles J. Hatem, MD
Mt. Auburn Hospital
Cambridge, Massachusetts

William R. Hazzard, MD
Bowman Gray School of Medicine
Winston-Salem, North Carolina

Cyril M. Hetsko, MD
Dean Clinic
Madison, Wisconsin

Robert S. Hillman, MD
University of Maryland School of
    Medicine
Baltimore, Maryland

Robert S. Hillman, MD
Maine Medical Center
Portland, Maine

E. Rodney Hornbake III, MD
North Shore Management Service
    Organization
Great Neck, New York

Holly J. Humphrey, MD
University of Chicago
Chicago, Illinois

Frank E. Iaquinta, MD
The Brooklyn Hospital Center
Brooklyn, New York

Michael B. Jacobs, MD
Stanford University Medical School
Stanford, California

A. H. Janoski, MD
Prudential Health Care Plan
Baltimore, Maryland

Norm Jensen, MD
University of Wisconsin—Madison
    Medical School
Madison, Wisconsin

Jerry C. Johnson, MD
University of Pennsylvania School of
    Medicine
Philadelphia, Pennsylvania

Warren D. Johnson, Jr., MD
Cornell University Medical College
New York, New York

Allen Kaplan, MD
SUNY—Health Sciences Center
Stony Brook, New York

Jerome P. Kassirer, MD
New England Journal of Medicine
Boston, Massachusetts

Paul Katz, MD
Monroe Community Hospital
Rochester, New York

Emmet B. Keeffe, MD
Stanford University Medical Center
Stanford, California

David Kemp, MD
Easton Hospital
Easton, Pennsylvania

Bryant D. Kendrick, D. Min.
Bowman Gray School of Medicine
Winston-Salem, North Carolina

Faroque A. Khan, MB
State University of New York at Stony
    Brook
East Meadow, New York

Marc J. Khan, MD
Tulane University Medical Center
New Orleans, Louisiana

Ronald Kindig, MD
Pacific Coast Internal Medicine
San Francisco, California

Mark A. Klempner, MD
Tufts–New England Medical Center
Boston, Massachusetts

Margo Krasnoff, MD
Buffalo, New York

Margaret Kreher, MD
Polyclinic Medical Center
Harrisburg, Pennsylvania

Frank J. Kroboth, MD
University of Pittsburgh School of
    Medicine
Pittsburgh, Pennsylvania

Paul A. Krusinski, MD
University of Vermont College of
    Medicine
Burlington, Vermont

Myron M. Laban, MD
Royal Oak, Mississippi

Michael A. LaCombe, MD
S. Paris, Maine

Thomas F. Lansdale III, MD
GBMC Healthcare, Inc.
Baltimore, Maryland

Richard C. Lavy, MD
University of Maryland
Annapolis, Maryland

Richard F. LeBlond, MD
University of Iowa Hospitals and Clinics
Iowa City, Iowa

Stephen S. Lefrak, MD
Jewish Hospital of St. Louis
St. Louis, Missouri

Matthew C. Leinung, MD
Albany Medical College
Albany, New York

Sandra Levinson, MD
Allegheny University Hospital
Philadelphia, Pennsylvania

David C. Lewis, MD
Brown University
Providence, Rhode Island

Matthew Liang, MD, MPH
Brigham and Women's Hospital
Boston, Massachusetts

Edgar Lichstein, MD
SUNY Health Science Center at Brooklyn
Brooklyn, New York

Mack Lipkin, Jr., MD
New York University Medical Center
New York, New York

Myron A. Lipkowitz, MD
Howell, New Jersey

J. Leonard Litchenfield, MD
Pikesville, Mississippi

John Luce, MD
San Francisco General Hospital
San Francisco, California

Robert Luke, MD
University of Cincinnati College of
    Medicine
Cincinnati, Ohio

Allan T. Luskin, MD
Dean Medicine Center
Sun Prairie, Wisconsin

Joanne Lynn, MD
Center to Improve Care of the Dying
Washington, D.C.

Thomas Mahl, MD
Veterans Affairs Medical Center
Buffalo, New York

Salvator Mangione, MD
Allegheny University Hospital
Philadelphia, Pennsylvania

Lyndon E. Mansfield, MD
University of Texas, El Paso
El Paso, Texas

Edward R. Marcantonio, MD
Brigham and Women's Hospital
Boston, Massachusetts

Joseph I. Matthews, MD
University of Colorado School of
    Medicine
Denver, Colorado

Robert J. Mayer, MD
Dana-Farber Cancer Institute
Boston, Massachusetts

John H. McConville, MD
York Hospital
York, Pennsylvania

Wayne McCormick, MD, MPH
Harborview Medical Center
Seattle, Washington

Sally McNagny, MD
Emory University School of Medicine
Atlanta, Georgia

Terrie Mendelson, MD
San Francisco Veterans Affairs Medical
  Center
San Francisco, California

David K. Meriney, MD
Upper Montclair, New Jersey

Catherine Messick, MD, MS
Bowman Gray School of Medicine
Winston-Salem, North Carolina

W. James Metzger, MD
Eastern Carolina University School of
  Medicine
Greenville, North Carolina

Robert M. Mile, MD
Lynchburg, Virginia

Gordon T. Moore, MD
Cambridge, Massachusetts

William P. Moran, MD, MS
Bowman Gray School of Medicine
Winston-Salem, North Carolina

Robert G. Narins, MD
Henry Ford Hospital
Detroit, Michigan

Thomas Nasco, MD
Thomas Jefferson University Hospital
Philadelphia, Pennsylvania

Eugene C. Nelson, DSc, MPH
Dartmouth-Hitchcock Medical Center
Lebanon, New Hampshire

David Nierenberg, MD
Dartmouth-Hitchcock Medical Center
Lebanon, New Hampshire

Edward J. O'Connell, MD
Mayo Clinic
Rochester, Minnesota

Eugene S. Ogrod III, MD
Sacramento Medical Foundation
Roseville, California

John M. O'Loughlin, MD
Lahey-Hitchcock Medical Center
Burlington, Massachusetts

Jerome Osheroff, MD
American College of Physicians
Philadelphia, Pennsylvania

Donald C. Overy, MD
American College of Cardiology
Bethesda, Massachusetts

Philip F. Panzarella, MD, MPH
Franklin Square Hospital Center
Baltimore, Maryland

Donna Parker, MD
University of Maryland School of
  Medicine
Baltimore, Maryland

Julie Patterson, MD
Dartmouth-Hitchcock Medical Center
Lebanon, New Hampshire

Steven Peitzman, MD
Allegheny University Hospital
Philadelphia, Pennsylvania

Col. Yancey Phillips, MD
Walter Reed Army Medical Center
Washington, D.C.

Allan Pont, MD
California Pacific Medical Center
San Francisco, California

Jay M. Portnoy, MD
Children's Mercy Hospital
Kansas City, Missouri

Gerald Posner, MD
Interfaith Medical Center
Brooklyn, New York

David W. Potts, MD
Greenville Hospital System
Greenville, South Carolina

Martin Raber, MD
M.D. Anderson Cancer Center
Houston, Texas

Eric C. Rackow, MD
St. Vincent's Hospital and Medical Center
New York, New York

Herbert Reynolds, MD
Pennsylvania State University College of
  Medicine
Hershey, Pennsylvania

P. Preston Reynolds, MD
Norfolk, Virginia

Sharon Riddler, MD
University of Pittsburgh
Pittsburgh, Pennsylvania

Michelle Roberts, MD
University of Pittsburgh Medical Center
Pittsburgh, Pennsylvania

W. Neal Roberts, MD
Medical College of Virginia
Richmond, Virginia

Murray M. Rosenberg, MD
New York, New York

Lawrence W. Roth, MD
San Jose, California

Judith Rubin, MD, MPH
University of Maryland
Baltimore, Maryland

Shaun Ruddy, MD
Medical College of Virginia
Richmond, Virginia

Gregory W. Rutecki, MD
Northeastern Ohio University
Affiliated Hospitals at Canton
Canton, Ohio

Merle Sande, MD
University of Utah School of Medicine
Salt Lake City, Utah

Karl J. Sandin, MD
Santa Barbara Rehabilitation Institute
Santa Barbara, California

Joseph Sapira, MD
Olivette, Missouri

Geraldine Schechter, MD
Veteran Affairs Medical Center
Washington, D.C.

Robert Scheig, MD
Buffalo General Hospital
Buffalo, New York

James Scheuer, MD
Albert Einstein College of Medicine of
  Yeshiva University
Bronx, New York

Daniel P. Schuster, MD
Barnes Hospital
St. Louis, Missouri

Richard J. Schuster, MD
Kettering Medical Center
Kettering, Ohio

Joanne Schwartzburg, MD
American Medical Association
Chicago, Illinois

Charles B. Seelig, MD, MS
Greenwich Hospital
Greenwich, Connecticut

Bernard P. Shangan, MD
Monmouth Medical Center
Long Branch, New Jersey

Jeanette Shorey, MD
Harvard Pilgrim Health Care
Boston, Massachusetts

David J. Shulkin, MD
University of Pennsylvania Medical Center
Philadelphia, Pennsylvania

Eugenia Siegler, MD
New York University School of Medicine
New York, New York

Lee S. Simon, MD
Beth Israel–Deaconess Medical Center
Boston, Massachusetts

Richard J. Simons, MD
Pennsylvania State College of Medicine
Hershey, Pennsylvania

Kelley M. Skeff, MD
Stanford University Medical Center
Stanford, California

C. Scott Smith, MD
Boise Veterans Affairs Medical Center
Boise, Idaho

David G. Smith, MD
Abington Memorial Hospital
Abington, Pennsylvania

Lawrence G. Smith, MD
Mt. Sinai Medical Center
New York, New York

Susan Smith, MD
McLaren Regional Medical Center
Flint, Michigan

William A. Sodeman, Jr., MD
Medical College of Ohio
Toledo, Ohio

Frederick Sparling, MD
University of North Carolina at Chapel
    Hill
Chapel Hill, North Carolina

David E. Steward, MD
Southern Illinois University School of
    Medicine
Springfield, Illinois

Brian Strom, MD, MPH
University of Pennsylvania School of
    Medicine
Philadelphia, Pennsylvania

Darryl Sue, MD
Harbor-UCLA Medical Center
Torrance, California

Gail Sullivan, MD
Veterans Affairs Medical Center
Newington, Connecticut

Martin I. Surks, MD
Montefiore Medical Center
Bronx, New York

Gerald S. Svedlow, MD
Professional Medical Associates
Santa Barbara, California

Richard Tannen, MD
University of Pennsylvania School of
    Medicine
Philadelphia, Pennsylvania

Ron Teichman, MD, MPH
Techman Occupational Health Associa-
    tion, Inc.
Baltimore, Maryland

Charles W. Thomas, MD
Medical College of Virginia
Richmond, Virginia

Patricia A. Thomas, MD
Johns Hopkins Bayview Medical Center
Baltimore, Maryland

Kate Thomson, MD
University of Medicine and Dentistry of
    New Jersey
Newark, New Jersey

Phillip P. Toskes, MD
Shands Hospital at the University of
    Florida
Gainesville, Florida

Gerald Turlo, MD
Detroit Medical Center
Detroit, Michigan

Sara E. Walker, MD
Harry S. Truman Memorial Veterans
    Affairs Hospital
Columbia, Missouri

Eleanor Z. Wallace, MD
Long Island Jewish Medical Center
Brooklyn, New York

Lisa B. Wallenstein, MD
Albert Einstein Medical Center
Philadelphia, Pennsylvania

Lila Wallis, MD
Cornell University
Naples, Florida

Stephen L. Wasserman, MD
University of California, San Diego,
    Medical Center
San Diego, California

Richard Weber, MD
National Jewish Center
Denver, Colorado

James P. Whalen, MD
University of Illinois at Chicago
Chicago, Illinois

Mark C. Wilson, MD, MPH
Bowman Gray School of Medicine
Winston-Salem, North Carolina

Charles J. Wolf, MD
Pennsylvania Hospital
Philadelphia, Pennsylvania

Susan D. Wolfsthal, MD
University of Maryland School of
    Medicine
Baltimore, Maryland

Toni Wymer, MD
Bowman Gray School of Medicine
Winston-Salem, North Carolina

Tadataka Yamada, MD
SmithKline Beecham Corporation
Philadelphia, Pennsylvania

Kevin Yingling, MD
Marshall University School of Medicine
Huntington, West Virginia

David I. Zolet, MD
Franklin Square Hospital Center
Baltimore, Maryland

Robert Zuckerman, MD
Harrisburg, Pennsylvania

INTRODUCTION

Internal medicine, the largest specialty within the medical profession, accounts for the greatest number of practicing generalist and subspecialist physicians. It trains more residents than any other branch of the profession and is responsible for a large share of student teaching at the preclinical and clinical levels. Internal medicine's contribution to biomedical and health services research is unsurpassed, and the large number of health policy and health industry leaders who are internists further substantiates its prominence. Yet internal medicine's importance does not rest with its present or past but with its future. It must therefore be a dynamic specialty that adapts continuously to new needs and environmental factors.

Like the medical profession as a whole, internal medicine finds itself buffeted by several forces. At times such as these, when the practices and products of the discipline are under scrutiny, internal medicine must be able to articulate its most important values and develop an organizing vision of what its future should include. For internal medicine, that organizing vision is embodied in its curriculum.

That internal medicine views its future through the lens of curriculum is quite apt. Internal medicine has always defined itself through the expertise of its practitioners and teachers, just as it has continuously reinvigorated itself through its trainees. It is impossible for internal medicine to retool for the challenges of the 21st century without first attending to the experiences offered through its graduate medical education programs.

The challenge of recasting internal medicine's curriculum was undertaken by the Federated Council for Internal Medicine, or FCIM, which brings together internal medicine's major organizations—its board, its college, its societies of practicing and academic generalists and subspecialists, and its organizations of chairs and program directors—into a single organization, to speak with a single voice. This book presents the work of FCIM's Task Force on Curriculum, but more accurately, it is the work of the internal medicine community, which has defined and articulated the competencies that physicians should attain—the skills, knowledge, and attitudes they should possess, and the experiences they should have—before they can be called internists.

This book has nine interrelated chapters. The first four chapters reflect the deliberative process by which the internal medicine community has developed this document. Chapter 1 describes the principal forces that shape medicine as a whole and internal medicine as a specialty. Internal medicine's expanding role in primary care, its internal and external relationships, and an appreciation of its mission appear here. What is internal medicine's mission and how best can it be accomplished are important questions that in the past may not have received the attention they deserved. Chapter 2 anticipates the role to be played by internal medicine in the 21st century. Here, too, appears a discussion of internal medicine's roots, hardy as ever, but in need of replanting in somewhat different soil. Emerging from Chapters 1 and 2 are a strong statement of internal medicine's values, a warning that internal medicine's practices must change, and ultimately, a justification for reconsidering how the internist should be trained.

Chapter 3 describes the potential significance of a curriculum and its utility as an instrument of change. Then to assist readers in understanding the function of this curricular resource document, Chapter 4 presents the Task Force's recommended approach to curriculum development in individual residency training programs.

The core content of this report appears in Chapters 5 and 6, beginning in Chapter 5 with the essential integrative aspects of internal medicine practice. Chapter 5 identifies the core values of effective internal medicine practitioners, how and where they practice, and the methods they employ as they utilize their knowledge and skills. Chapter 6 contains the competencies of 23 topics of internal medicine; these competencies are collectively the knowledge base that all general internists should have.

Chapter 7 presents the residency learning experience. It includes descriptions of rotations, or learning experiences, and didactic programs. These descriptions capture much of what makes internal medicine training special, separate from the competencies it conveys. Some of the described learning experiences, such as the intensive care unit and ward rotations, are familiar; others may be novel and should stimulate departments to develop new learning venues and new approaches to graduate medical education. Chapter 8 provides an overview of didactic teaching methods and shows how to use these methods to teach the competencies.

Chapter 9 addresses issues of implementation and organization and describes how this book can facilitate curriculum development at the institutional level. This book specifies competencies and describes experiences, but it cannot stipulate the venue, sequence, or length of those experiences. Each program must make these decisions for itself, so that it can make the best use of its resources and identify the additional resources needed to achieve its goals. Thus, Chapters 5 through 9 provide a process by which program directors can adapt the curricular goals and objectives of this report for local use. The book ends with Chapter 10, which presents final recommendations and future directions.

Readers have every right to ask, "What is the intended result of this book, and how will it shape the ever-changing world of internal medicine's residency education?" We present it with a sense of optimism and, indeed, excitement that internal medicine has at last defined the goals of its residency education. But the actual impact of this report depends on how program directors use the competency lists to shape their program's curriculum. The competency lists provide a stimulus for residency programs in internal medicine to assess their individual curricula and to identify areas in need of change, and the methods by which to bring about those changes. This resource document also has a public purpose. It describes the content of internal medicine and should allow the public and private sectors to attain a clearer understanding of what internists do.

This report is not the last word on the curriculum of internal medicine. It is a dynamic document that internal medicine must revisit and revise. The Task Force would like to see this resource document updated as often as necessary but no less frequently than every 5 years. Internal medicine will renew itself through its curriculum. As an exploration of internal medicine's identity, the curriculum is a critical means of maintaining the preeminence of internal medicine training programs and the excellence of its patient care.

The Report of the Task Force is internal medicine's effort to anticipate the knowledge, skills, and attitudes that internists will need to practice in the future. It is a tool to help individual program directors to assess how well their programs meet today's needs and then to make changes through the vehicle of curriculum.

A discipline that defines itself by listing the knowledge and skills of its practitioners does so at the risk that some readers will misunderstand the purpose of the report. To avoid this outcome, the Task Force here describes the intent of its report:

> This report is a resource to help an individual residency program to design a curriculum that fits its resources and responds to the aspirations of its residents and faculty. It helps programs to improve through the medium of curriculum.

In the process of discussing this report, the organizations that represent internal medicine have spoken with one voice in agreeing with the FCIM Task Force about what the report is *not*:

- The report is not a "one-size-fits-all" curriculum that FCIM is mandating for all residency programs.
- The report is not a list of requirements by which accrediting organizations, such as the Residency Review Committee for Internal Medicine, will judge a residency program.

CHAPTER 1

THE FORCES SHAPING INTERNAL MEDICINE

IMPLICATIONS FOR INTERNAL MEDICINE RESIDENCY TRAINING

Internal medicine has had a long and distinguished record as an intellectual discipline dedicated to clinical observation, discovery of new knowledge, and the application of this knowledge to human disease. For the entire 20th century, training has centered on the hospital, in which the sickest patients in the community have received care and young physicians have learned the skills of diagnosis and treatment and how to apply their knowledge of the scientific basis of medicine. This hospital-based tradition helped to define the role of the internist-consultant who provided advice to general practitioners and to surgical colleagues. The internist became the consummate diagnostician and the physician best equipped to handle the complex problems of sick adults.

Until the late 20th century, many internists practiced in large urban areas and aligned themselves with teaching hospitals. These internists were primary care physicians who also did consultation, particularly in the hospital. In smaller communities, internists were consultants in all aspects of internal medicine and often were the only physicians, besides surgeons, who had any advanced training.

Beginning in the 1960s, two emerging forces changed this model of internal medicine practice. The first was the rapid growth of internal medicine subspecialty practice, which reduced the demand for medical consultation by general internists. The second force was society's desire to control medical costs. The subsequent emergence of managed care and the role of the primary care physician led to a reduction in hospital care, which had been a strength of internal medicine practice, and an increase in ambulatory care. Office-based primary care became the focus of most general internists.

Other forces are emerging in the 1990s. Large corporations are organizing health care delivery systems in which physicians have less and less control of their practice environment. Physicians' compensation is increasingly dependent on their ability to control costs. Reimbursement is declining. Legislators are questioning the public's obligation to support medical training, and market forces are beginning to reshape the physician workforce. These forces are substantially changing the face of American medical practice.

The outcome of these changes is not entirely predictable. Medical practice in the United States has distinctive regional patterns, determined by population demographics, the number of physicians, culture, and local economics. In addition, the explosive growth of knowledge of basic mechanisms of disease will change medical practice and its economics as discoveries occur in such areas as AIDS, cancer, diabetes, and heart disease. Finally, there is public backlash against the extreme manifestations of corporate business values in medical care.

In the midst of uncertainty and yet certain of change, internal medicine must reexamine its postgraduate training. Internal medicine residency must provide internists with skills and knowledge that fit society's health care needs and that build on internal medicine's many strengths. The foundation of residency training should be a curriculum, which is a formal description of the content of training. The curriculum must be flexible enough to accommodate diverse career pathways for internists. The remainder of this chapter describes some of the external forces that affect American medicine. An internal medicine curriculum must respond to these forces.

1. Medical care will continue to move out of the hospital and into other settings.

The most costly component of medical care is hospitalization. Both the federal government and private health maintenance organizations (HMOs) have introduced changes designed to reduce expenditures for hospitalized patients. Fixed payments per diagnosis and HMO preauthorization of hospital care—arrangements that have been in place for over a decade—have reduced both hospital costs and inpatient utilization to among the lowest of the industrialized nations.

With the success of these arrangements, patients are seldom admitted to the hospital to establish a diagnosis. Better imaging technology and procedure units for ambulatory patients have shifted the locus of most diagnostic workups to the ambulatory setting. People enter the hospital when they become too ill to remain at home or require the technical content of care that only hospitals provide. Patients with some disorders, such as chronic congestive heart failure and many types of pulmonary and gastrointestinal disease, are admitted only when they become so ill that they require treatment that cannot be accomplished safely at home. Ambulatory patients who require hospitalization stay only briefly for specific services such as chemotherapy or cardiac catheterization, with their care often directed by the standardized procedures of critical pathways. Technology breakthroughs, such as videoscopic surgery, will continue to reduce the amount of time that patients spend in the hospital.

The shift to the ambulatory setting has already influenced internal medicine practice and training. Internists who previously had many inpatients now typically have only a few. Often, they have no one in the hospital. More and more, one's inpatient service consists of patients who are critically ill or dying and who represent a very small, though still very important, proportion of internal medicine practice. Instead, most internists have a large panel of patients whose medical problems they can usually manage in the ambulatory setting. Reduction in hospital care has created new venues in which the general internist must now be proficient, such as the home, the nursing home, and the rehabilitation facility. Feedback from internists who have just started practice suggests that residency training has not kept pace with these changes.

The shift from the inpatient to the outpatient arena has already had major effects on education. First, housestaff on inpatient rotations no longer see many conditions and diseases that were common in the hospital setting, such as stable coronary disease, occult gastrointestinal bleeding, and uncomplicated peptic ulcer disease. Second, reduced length of stay in the hospital allows little time for trainees to observe and study patients, as was the norm a generation ago. Currently, many patients enter the hospital with a diagnosis, treatment plan, and targeted length of stay.

Because of these changes, internal medicine training must shift to the ambulatory setting. There formidable challenges await. Unlike hospital-based training, each learning opportunity, each act of caring for the patient requires faculty supervision, which means that education in the ambulatory setting is expensive. General internal medicine office practice affords limited exposure to many diseases that internists must be able to recognize and manage. There are fewer opportunities to learn from colleagues' patients in office practice than in the hospital, where cross-coverage provided by inpatient teams provides many learning opportunities. Finally, managed care places a premium on efficiency and reducing overhead. Teaching is inefficient and adds overhead. This economic reality has affected inpatient learning and will pose an even greater threat to the educational mission in the ambulatory setting.

2. The role of the primary care physician will expand.

As inpatient practice has diminished, the general internist's role as a primary care physician has increased at the expense of the consultant role. This outcome is the result of several factors, the most compelling of which is the unparalleled growth of medical subspecialties over the last two decades. The expansion brought sophisticated consultation within easy reach of community practitioners, reducing the consultant role for general internists. Simultaneously, the growth of health insurance, particularly in managed care, created a demand for well-trained primary care physicians who could manage their patients with less reliance on consultants. This force is likely to persist indefinitely.

In most urban and suburban areas, the typical general internist is a primary care physician who seeks consultation from colleagues but does little consulting. Most clinical activity is in office-based practice where health insurance structures the economic incentives. In fee-for-service care, practice is volume-driven; in capitated care, the focus is efficiency and preventive care.

The primary care internist is in great demand and will likely be the most common career pathway for general internists. Primary practice requires broad skills in areas that have received little attention in internal medicine training (e.g., behavioral disorders, musculoskeletal injuries, women's health, and prevention). The challenge to internal medicine educators is to incorporate these topics into the curriculum and still produce internists who can fulfill internal medicine's essential role in the community: to care for very sick patients whose problems require skill in all of the organ-based specialties. Physicians who embody this traditional strength of internal medicine and have the new ambulatory skills will always have a special role in the community.

3. The practice of medicine will become more highly organized.

The residency curriculum is developing against the backdrop of the industrialization of American medicine. For-profit and not-for-profit entities are acquiring hospitals, organizing physicians, and developing insurance products. Nationally, the practice of medicine is being organized into large, vertically integrated physician groups. General internists will increasingly practice in such groups, which are themselves part of larger integrated health systems. The forms of practice include a staff-model HMO, in which the internist is a member of a multispecialty group practice, and membership in a group of independent physicians who share economic risk through managed care contracts. There is growing evidence that these practice groups are more cost-effective than traditional forms of practice organization.

These trends mean that physicians must now be prepared to function in teams whose success will be measured by medical outcomes, cost, and patient satisfaction. Physicians will increasingly assume responsibility for large groups of patients and populations through contractual relationships with managed care organizations. Payment through capitation means that internists' income will depend on success in keeping costs under control. Internists will therefore need training in medical economics, practice management, quality improvement, and medical informatics.

The reorganization of medical practice means that internal medicine training is undergoing a philosophic shift. Traditionally, internists have focused on the individual patient and the intellectual exercise of precise diagnosis and treatment. The importance of these priorities is undiminished, but educators are learning to balance them against the new perspectives of population-based risk, prevention, and living with diagnostic uncertainty. Many program directors are arranging rotations to provide experience in managed care in large health care delivery organizations.

4. Medical knowledge will continue to expand rapidly.

The science of medicine—including biology, therapeutics, epidemiology, technology, and health care economics—is growing at an unprecedented rate. As medicine stands on the threshold of new discoveries about the human genome, fundamental approaches to disease may change radically within a generation.

Internists' ability to provide a fresh perspective on diverse patients, each one unique and complex, derives in large part from reasoning from basic principles of biology and pathophysiology. This historic strength of internal medicine will be increasingly difficult to sustain in today's learning environment. The rapid pace of care in all settings leaves too little time for contemplation, speculation, and discourse. Physicians in the clinic formulate diagnostic hypotheses but often must leave the testing of these hypotheses to physicians who work in the hospital. Hospital-based physicians seldom see the long-term outcome of treatments that they initiate. The rapid pace of care in the ambulatory setting poses a particularly sharp challenge to learning the scientific basis of clinical phenomena. Nonetheless, we must find a way.

Internal medicine has been strong in part because it emphasizes the scientific basis of medicine and evidence-based medical practice. These fundamental skills prepare the internist to learn over a professional lifetime, continuously refreshing and updating the knowledge acquired in residency. Medical informatics is an important skill in dealing with the expanding knowledge base of internal medicine practice to patient care. In the future, physicians may learn to apply basic biology to medical practice by using the computer on their office desktop to access information that is pertinent to a current patient.

5. The growth of the elderly population in the United States will strongly influence medical practice.

The elderly population in the United States is growing rapidly. Advancing age increases the probability that patients will have several chronic diseases. Understanding the complex interaction of these diseases and their management is the internist's core skill. As the population ages, the internist's role in medical care will grow. Consequently, experience in geriatric care in all of its settings will become increasingly important during residency training. Currently, many older persons reside in nursing homes, life-care facilities, or other such institutions, making these venues important for practice and thus for training.

6. Internists will continue to have a spectrum of career opportunities.

While internists will be in demand as primary care physicians, they will have other career opportunities. The design of a curriculum must take into account the full spectrum of the future internist's career options.

General internists are not all alike. In rural areas, there are relatively few subspecialists, and general internists perform subspecialty consultation and do procedures that would be the exclusive province of board-certified subspecialists in more densely populated areas. There is a trend toward internists specializing in hospital practice. Some insurers and health systems are discovering that primary care physicians who are heavily committed to ambulatory practice are not efficient in hospital care or, conversely, that caring for patients in the hospital interferes with the efficiency of office practice. In response, some organizations are recruiting internists to provide hospital care for patients of primary care physicians who wish to specialize in ambulatory practice. The internist is comfortable in the hospital setting and can manage patients with multiple medical problems without unnecessary consultation.

Many internists will continue to choose careers in the medical subspecialties. Considerable evidence indicates that the number of subspecialists in practice now is adequate or excessive relative to the needs of the American people for general internists. However, market and educational forces should eventually redress this imbalance. There will ultimately be a reduced but appropriate demand for medical subspecialists. The demand for subspecialists' expertise in scientific investigation and teaching the application of basic science to medical practice will continue.

7. Economic forces will change the structure of graduate medical education.

The continuing debate over the size and composition of the physician workforce has centered on whether the number of training positions in subspecialties and even in primary care is excessive. In its quest to balance the federal budget, Congress has targeted public funding for medical education. Health insurance companies have resisted calls for all payers to share in the cost of graduate medical education. The convergence of these forces will affect graduate medical education, but there are other important influences at play.

Graduate medical education will become more expensive as it moves into the ambulatory setting. On the inpatient teaching service, faculty must supervise residents and be involved directly in patient care, but their involvement is leveraged by the presence of housestaff who spend long hours caring for patients in the hospital. Now, as medical education moves to the ambulatory arena, trainees will cover inpatients less frequently, and hospitals must find relatively expensive substitutes. Furthermore, outpatient faculty must spend much more time in supervision relative to the inpatient teaching service. The increased cost of ambulatory teaching, the attendant curricular changes, and the shift to ambulatory teaching mean that the residents' education needs are increasingly taking priority over the hospital's service needs.

The outcome of these economic forces and education trends will be the reorganization of academic centers and their residency programs. Some programs will dissolve because the sponsoring hospital cannot afford them. As hospitals merge and reduce bed capacity, they will reduce the size of their housestaff training programs. Large health systems may tailor graduate medical education programs to meet their need for a steady flow of well-trained graduate physicians to work in their organizations. Success in postgraduate medical education, like success in medical practice, may favor larger organizations that have the resources to support education.

While these economic trends should not affect curricular content, they may influence the way in which programs implement their curricula. For economic and logistic reasons, internal medicine training programs may have to share such resources as ambulatory facilities, clinical faculty, and patients. Cooperation between institutions and disciplines may help programs to preserve their educational mission in today's challenging external environment.

CHAPTER 2

THE GENERAL INTERNIST FOR THE 21ST CENTURY

SETTING OUR SIGHTS—AND OUR CURRICULUM— FOR THE YEARS AHEAD

Those who write their institution's curriculum for internal medicine residency training must understand the roles of general internists and their relationship to other generalist physicians. Reconsideration of a curriculum is an opportunity to explore the common ground internists share with other primary care physicians and to identify the attributes that distinguish the general internist from other providers of comprehensive care for adults.

In developing this curricular resource document, the Federated Council for Internal Medicine (FCIM) Task Force on the Internal Medicine Residency Curriculum used the vision of the future general internist, as defined by the American College of Physicians (ACP) Task Force on the Physician Workforce, which is summarized below.

Today's General Internist: Similarities to Other Generalist Physicians

Like other generalists, the general internist is a primary care physician who establishes initial contact with adult patients from adolescence to very old age and provides comprehensive and continuing care. Although some general internists are hospital-based consultants who focus on patients referred by family practitioners for hospitalization or office consultation, most assume a central role in primary care.

Primary care physicians evaluate and manage all aspects of illness—biomedical and psychosocial—in the patient. The focus on reducing health care costs, the dominant feature of health care in the 1990s, has placed a premium on physicians who can manage most of their patients' problems without obtaining consultation.

Today's physicians spend many of their office hours on prevention, early detection of disease, and health promotion. Disease prevention requires knowledge and judgment to determine when a patient's level of risk requires additional screening, counseling, or prophylaxis.

Primary care physicians also act as patients' guides and advocates in a complex health care environment. The complexity of today's health care system intimidates many patients and families. Other patients are victims of fragmented care, which managed care, with its emphasis on the primary physician's role as care manager, may help to ameliorate. A key role for primary care physicians is to organize their patients' care and help them gain access to the care they need. Many very old patients have physical or intellectual disabilities and greatly need vigorous advocacy from their physician.

Today's General Internist: Distinctive Features

A distinguishing trait of general internists is their expertise in managing patients with advanced illness and diseases of several organ systems. The internist's distinctive role in the community is to care for the sickest patients and most complex cases, often at the request of another physician. Learning to manage sick patients efficiently immediately before, during, and after surgery and during and after hospitalization has always been the focal point of the internist's training. Until recently, it was possible to admit patients to the hospital in order to take a contemplative approach to a difficult problem, but now the internist must display the same diagnostic acumen and therapeutic ingenuity in the ambulatory setting.

People are living longer, and many face a long, gradual decline that poses many diagnostic and therapeutic challenges. Patients with advanced, chronic disease require medical knowledge, judgment, and experience, as well as great patience and skill in working with community resources. The internist has never had a greater opportunity to help sick people maintain good function and find dignity and tranquillity during the last months of life.

The general internist may also serve as a consultant when patients have difficult undifferentiated problems or well-defined problems to which the general internist can bring special expertise. For years, "diagnostician" was almost synonymous with "internist," reflecting the internist's key role in the professional community as a solver of difficult diagnostic problems. As explained in Chapter 1, that role has been diminished by the growth of subspecialty medicine, especially in large group practices and metropolitan areas.

However, the general internist remains the best consultant for a large number of patients with undifferentiated diagnostic problems. As the medical education system produces fewer subspecialists, general internists may enjoy a resurgence as consultants. Referrals between general internist and internist-subspecialist may flow in both directions.

The Future General Internist

The general internist of the future is likely to differ in important ways from today's general internist. In addition to mastering a greater breadth of skills, as exemplified by the competency lists in this report, general internists will need to play several different roles. The first two, resource manager and clinical information manager, are in response to changes in the medical care environment. The third role, the generalist with an area of special expertise, is not new but may become more prominent.

Resource Manager

The future general internist must be a resource manager who, familiar with the sciences of clinical epidemiology and decision making, brings a thoughtful, lean style of practice to patient evaluation and management. Primary care physicians must reconcile two strong forces: the wishes of the patient and the limits on health care resources. Clinical epidemiology, decision analysis, and medical ethics offer principles that can help the physician serve the patient's interests in the context of resource constraints. Research on the application of these principles to patient care has yielded many practical contributions to clinical medicine. For example, per capita utilization of some procedures varies four- to eightfold among different hospital referral areas. Clinical epidemiology, decision analysis, and medical ethics can help physicians determine the appropriate rate of utilization. The internist who can apply the lessons of these disciplines to everyday practice will be a leader in defining standards of care in the community.

Clinical Information Manager

The future general internist must be a clinical information manager who can take full advantage of electronically stored data and who can communicate using current technology. Modern information technology is improving medical practice. The desktop computer speeds access to patient data and medical knowledge. Decision analyses accessed by computer can play a role in difficult decisions. Physicians will need to be able to analyze electronically stored practice data to understand and improve their practice. Electronic mail, two-way interactive video, and long-distance access to electronically stored patient records will improve patient care and enhance enjoyment of practice. Internists in training must master the use of this information technology.

Generalist and Specialist

The future generalist internist must be a generalist in outlook, and at the same time many will wish to possess skills that respond to the needs of a particular care environment. For example, in many rural areas with limited access to subspecialists, general internists may be expert in a specific area of internal medicine and may be the first line of referral care in that subspecialty. Many perform invasive diagnostic procedures that are the exclusive province of subspecialist internists in urban practice. Patients in rural communities served by such internists get in-depth care in an organ-based subspecialty of internal medicine. The need for on-site subspecialty care by general internists with an area of special expertise may grow if the United States moves toward training only enough subspecialists to satisfy the needs of referral centers.

Many trainees use time during residency to prepare for a niche in the community practice of general internal medicine. They learn the cognitive content of a subspecialty field, obtain extra experience in diagnosis and management, and acquire skills to perform some necessary procedures. Some focus on traditional, organ system–based subspecialties and acquire their special expertise either during residency or by returning for additional training after entering practice. Others obtain extra training in the "new subspecialties" of internal medicine, which include geriatric medicine, adolescent medicine, care of medical illness during pregnancy, substance abuse, women's health issues, and sports medicine. Expertise in these topics will continue to be valuable in community practice, whether in a rural locale or in a large suburban or urban managed care practice.

The capacity of the general internist to practice according to the needs of his or her environment has implications for training, day-to-day practice, and the shape of the physician workforce. Housestaff programs, which have heretofore focused on teaching the in-depth reasoning required of an internist and the care of complicated, hospitalized patients, must now also provide learning opportunities for the large fraction of residents who will become self-reliant primary care physicians. The competencies described in this report delineate the breadth and depth of internal medicine.

CHAPTER 3

WHAT IS A CURRICULUM AND WHY IS IT IMPORTANT?

Until a few years ago, residency programs in internal medicine did not have a written curriculum. Nonetheless, the leaders who defined the standards of internal medicine considered the training more than sufficient and felt that the graduates were well prepared for internal medicine practice. Why does internal medicine now concern itself with curriculum? Several reasons can be cited, but none is more compelling than the need to assure that clinical training is relevant to practice. As previous chapters indicate, the gap separating clinical training and practice has widened and appears unlikely to close without bona fide educational reform. An explicit curriculum is the blueprint for education reform.

Ours is not the first decade of this century to appreciate a mismatch between clinical training and practice. Contemporary challenges parallel closely those faced by medical education reformers at the turn of the century. Before Osler installed the first clinical clerkship and then the first hospital-based residency at Johns Hopkins in the 1890s, clinical training took place in amphitheaters; hospitals seldom accommodated trainees. But after Osler, inspired by his success and guided by their own training in more advanced institutions in Europe, medical education reformers of the early 20th century embraced a new vision that insisted on direct involvement with patients. This vision ultimately led medical schools and teaching hospitals to form liaisons that met everyone's needs until the present time. Now, as we have seen in these pages, program directors and departmental chairs no longer can rely on the hospital ward to provide residents with reliable preparation for practice, and graduate medical education is shifting to ambulatory settings. As new settings require new educational plans, interest in curriculum rises.

Interest, however, does not always go hand in hand with clarity and consensus. Part of the confusion surrounding curriculum stems from differences in people's conceptions of curriculum. Is curriculum a list of competencies—the knowledge, skills, and attitudes that internists should have—or is it the sequence and mix of training experiences that enable residents to acquire these competencies? Or might there be a way to join these two models of curriculum? In this report, the Task Force acknowledges attempts to chart the relationship between competencies and learning experiences. In one sense, the competencies justify the experiences: Because internists need to know how to evaluate a thyroid nodule, they should spend time in thyroid clinic, or wherever patients with a thyroid nodule are found. But in another sense, the experiences of clinical practice define the competencies: Because general internists work in office settings, they must be able to evaluate heart murmurs; so they should be competent in cardiac auscultation. A graduate medical education curriculum, therefore, must link competencies and experiences. A curriculum should enable learners to develop competencies, and it should specify those competencies in a way that program directors can use to shape the learning experiences in their institutions. Ultimately, the curriculum of internal medicine will define our discipline, by specifying the knowledge base and skill that we require and the settings in which we can practice effectively.

A curriculum is principally pedagogic, but it also has administrative, financial, and political implications. Administratively, a curriculum may call for new or different relationships within and between institutions. For example, it may be difficult to teach the principles of managed care in institutions that bar residents from managed care practice. The feasibility of teaching sports medicine depends on the cooperation of the sports medicine clinic. The Task Force has noted the substantial cost of shifting education from the hospital to the outpatient setting. Implementing a curriculum generates costs, and public funding for graduate medical education is precarious. Curricular change based on this report will challenge academic medical centers' commitment to education. At the very least, creating a new curriculum will stimulate institutions to think about discarding outdated models of training and consider new arrangements for sharing or defraying the costs of education.

Politically, a curriculum stakes out the boundaries of a specialty vis-à-vis other specialties and subspecialties. Throughout the development of consensus around this resource document for curriculum design, internists have tried to characterize general internal medicine and then have asked what distinguishes it from other primary care specialties and from internal medicine subspecialties. At the very least, the boundaries of the field should become evident by closely examining the competencies of the general internist as internists have defined them. Within these competency lists can be found internal medicine's distinctive, principal role in adult primary care.

In the final analysis, this resource document and the competency-based curricula it engenders will be judged by their effectiveness as instruments of change. Faculty, residents, program directors, and chairs can measure its worth across several dimensions. Will it facilitate the shift from inpatient to clinically relevant outpatient teaching? Will it affect the balance point between service and education? Will it provide leverage for departments to augment institutional commitments and resources? Will it affect the blueprint for certification of the internist? And will it alter the public and professional image of internal medicine as a field and the medical students' perceptions of general internal medicine as a career? In these outcomes will lie the answers to the questions, what is a curriculum and why is it important?

CHAPTER 4

THE VALUES, ASSUMPTIONS, AND METHODS OF THIS PROJECT

This project began in the late fall of 1993 when the FCIM Council convened a task force to reconsider internal medicine training in the light of today's practice environment. The task force members included representatives of each of the six FCIM organizations and two at-large education experts. The American College of Physicians Education Division provided staff support for the project. At its first meeting, the Task Force heard from general internists who represented a broad spectrum of general internal medicine practice, including urban, rural, private, and managed care practices. From these discussions, from the report of the ACP Task Force on the Physician Workforce, and from other background reading material, the Task Force conceptualized the general internist of the future. Concurrently, the Task Force tried to articulate the values of internal medicine, as reflected in practicing internists and in their training. The Task Force came to consensus on the following principles:

1. *Training should support diverse career paths.* A new approach to curriculum design should support one of internal medicine's historic strengths, the diversity of career opportunity for the internist. Some internists may be office-based practitioners; others may work exclusively in hospitals. In rural areas, internists may serve as first-line subspecialists and consultants. Training should provide a foundation of skills and discipline that would allow internists to be successful in any of these roles.

2. *Residency is part of a continuum of learning internal medicine.* Undergraduate medical education and continuing medical education must complement residency training.

3. *Internal medicine should reaffirm the importance of in-depth knowledge of the diseases of organ systems while acknowledging the importance of knowledge in new areas.* There must be more emphasis, not less, on acquiring a firm understanding of basic science in medicine. This traditional strength of internal medicine can be the foundation upon which to base scientific understanding of the new domains of the internist (e.g., orthopedics, women's health).

4. *Learning that used to occur with hospitalized patients will take place with these patients in the ambulatory arena.* This change may involve learning in subspecialty clinics as well as expansion of continuity ambulatory practice experience.

5. *Mastery of integrative disciplines and clinical competencies can occur together.* Learning how to reason from clinical data to scientific understanding and thence to disease recognition and treatment is as much the cornerstone of internal medi-

cine training as the tradition of using ethical, humanistic, and professional principles to guide our actions. Acquiring the broad range of competencies of internal medicine need not occur at the expense of developing skill in the integrative disciplines. In reality, every patient, no matter what their chief complaint, is an opportunity to extend one's mastery of these disciplines while simultaneously extending one's breadth of knowledge of disease and pathophysiology.

6. *Internal medicine practice has changed and so should its curriculum.* Competencies that have not been part of traditional training are now essential and should be part of the curriculum.

The Working Assumptions of the Task Force

After considering several different approaches to the development of an internal medicine residency curriculum, the Task Force agreed on the following assumptions:

1. The Task Force should focus on helping program directors to design a curriculum for the future general internist. Not all residents will become general internists, and the design of the residency curriculum should take into account the career aspirations and learning needs of the residents. Many programs will decide that all residents should acquire the competencies of the general internist. All of the residents in these programs will have the same set of required rotations. Residents will reveal the diversity of their career goals in their choice of elective experiences. Some programs may decide to have clear-cut tracks with different sets of required experiences for subspecialty-bound residents and future general internists. For logistical considerations, even these programs are likely to have a core content common to both tracks, and program directors may find this report useful in designing the core experience. The Task Force did not undertake to advise these program directors on what to put in the core curriculum and what to leave out. Each program director faces a different set of constraints and will base decisions about content on the resources and the mission of the individual program.

2. The Task Force would take a competency-based approach to curriculum design. Specifying the desired characteristics, or competencies, of the learner is a time-honored approach to curriculum design. The Task Force reviewed curricula from internal medicine and other disciplines and used some of them as models.

3. The Task Force would specify desirable competencies for general internists. The Task Force identified the topics of internal medicine education and then listed the competencies of each topic. The topics include the traditional medical subspecialties, new clinical areas (such as adolescent medicine), and the integrative disciplines (skills, such as epidemiology and medical ethics as well as humanism, professionalism, and general clinical skills, that apply to all medical encounters). The Task Force offers these topics and competencies as a resource

from which individual program directors will draw as they design a curriculum suited to their local environments. The report of the Task Force is a resource. It is not a prescriptive "one-size-fits-all" curriculum.

4. The FCIM curriculum report would describe in general terms the training experiences—the rotations, continuity practices, and didactic exercises—that constitute the core of a prototype residency training experience. In an individual program, the actual descriptions of these experiences would follow from the competencies that the program director assigned to each of these venues of learning.

5. Mastery of a competency requires repeated exposures to patients. The optimal number of exposures depends on the complexity of the competency and its frequency in medical practice.

6. The competencies that a trainee could acquire in a learning experience or rotation should shape its structure and content. The number of patients required to achieve a competency and the density of such patients in an educational setting should be important factors in determining the length of time in that setting.

7. The role of the FCIM Task Force would be to create a process that would facilitate curriculum design that would occur locally, that would be directed by individual program directors, and that would be consistent with local resources and requirements.

8. The Task Force would strive for consensus. It would directly involve the stakeholders in residency training in the process of developing and reviewing competency lists. These stakeholders include program directors, practitioners, generalists, subspecialists, and residents.

9. The Task Force assumed that the length of residency training is not likely to increase beyond 36 months.

The Task Force identified a working group that took principal responsibility for the project. The Task Force as a whole met periodically to review progress and advise on the direction of the project. Individual Task Force members had responsibility for choosing members of their organizations to participate in drafting the competency lists.

The Competencies of Internal Medicine

Guided by these principles, the working group identified topics of internal medicine, the competencies within those topics, and the types of learning experiences (venues) that together constitute the core of this resource document. Competencies in the integrative disciplines are presented first, followed by the clinical areas.

Each competency list represents a consensus of internists. At least two individuals, each a member of one of the organizations comprising FCIM, wrote a competency list using a template prepared by the Task Force working group. A member of the Task Force working group synthesized each set of lists into one. Three-person review teams, each led by an APDIM program director and usually including a general internist who had recently entered practice and a subspecialist in the pertinent discipline, reviewed each competency list and suggested revisions. The working group of the Task Force did the final editing in response to suggestions from the reviewers and from the FCIM organizations.

Learning Venues

The learning venues include the inpatient ward rotation, inpatient and office-based subspecialty rotation, ambulatory care clinic, emergency room, and community-based practice. The description of each venue includes its educational rationale, required resources, and logistic considerations. Some of the less familiar venues, such as home care and nursing home rotations, required additional description. After the learning venues, the report presents recommendations for shaping didactic programs.

Relating Competencies to Venues

A fundamental premise of this approach to curriculum design is that program directors should assign time in a learning venue in proportion to its educational value as determined by the competencies that residents can attain therein. A corollary of this premise is that the faculty of individual rotations accept responsibility for providing access to patients and other learning experiences that residents need in order to acquire specific competencies. To facilitate this process of assigning competencies to venues, the Task Force has supplied worksheets for each competency list. For the integrative disciplines, the worksheets allow program directors to relegate individual competencies to specific clinical rotations or to structured didactic programs. For the clinical areas, the worksheets list the competencies but leave it to the program director to endorse or revise the priority rating that the Task Force assigned to each competency, to add competencies, and then to assign each competency to a venue or rotation. The worksheets contain blank columns and rows to encourage program directors to tailor the worksheet to the character of the individual program. The Task Force expects that program directors will work with the faculty of individual rotations to make these assignments. In the process, program directors will learn about the educational value of existing venues; they may identify needs for new venues; and at the very least, they will form opinions about which components of their program's total curriculum should occur in each rotation. We describe this process further in Chapters 5, 6, 8, and 9.

Review and Comment

The final step in the development of this resource document was a review and commentary by the organizations that make up FCIM. This process began at a stakeholders' conference. Representatives from all FCIM organizations attended this conference, reviewed the entire report of the Task Force, reached consensus on many issues, and endorsed the approach that the Task Force developed to facilitate curriculum change in individual programs. Subsequently, many individuals and organizations have reviewed the Task Force report and offered suggestions. The working group of the Task Force responded to these suggestions by making substantial revisions to the report. The process of review, comment, and revision continued as the organizations that compose FCIM reviewed the Task Force report. The governing council of each of the organizations endorsed this report, and in November 1996, the FCIM Council unanimously endorsed the report.

Chapter 5

The Integrative Disciplines

The student must see, and hear, and feel for himself. The hue of the complexion, the feel of the skin, the luster and languor of the eye, the throbbing of the pulse and palpitations of the heart. Where can these be learned but at the bedside of the sick?

These words of Samuel Bard, MD, are over 100 years old, yet they are timeless. Physicians have always recognized the importance of learning from patients, under the supervisory eye of experienced clinicians, in realistic settings. Bard emphasized learning about disease—the languor of the eye, the feel of the pulse. But we wonder if he would not agree that there is another reason for educating students and residents in realistic settings, a reason that overshadows even learning about disease: learning to become a physician.

Learning to become a physician requires acculturation and socialization, irreplaceable outcomes of learning in realistic settings. Medical educators recognize that the actual outcomes are not always desirable. Several authors have commented that residency training can have a dehumanizing effect, that it can do more harm than good. However, that outcome is not a necessary consequence of practice-based training; more likely it reflects a training environment that is unprofessional or inhumane. In fact, the shift of training from inpatient to ambulatory settings presents an opportunity to avoid some of the harshness associated with training environments of the past.

As this shift is about to occur, program directors should pause and reflect on the specific lessons they would have their residents learn from both hospital-based and outpatient rotations. Knowledge of disease, in the sense identified by Bard, is a given. But here we ask, "What else? What else about the practice of internal medicine would we have our residents acquire in the context of patient care?"

The question deserves a thoughtful response. In several ways it asks, "What besides their knowledge of disease do the best internists invoke as they practice their profession?" The answers may be found in those hard-to-define aspects of internal medicine that internists render as part of every patient encounter.

The Task Force approached this challenge in two ways. First, we put this question to several expert internists. Specifically, we asked them to identify those difficult-to-measure properties of the expert internist that might be overlooked after biomedical knowledge and skills are presented in organ-specific competency lists. Their answers form a construct that we call "physicianship." It defines the difference between the expert internist and the journeyman practitioner. The development of physicianship is a complement to Bard's rationale for education in the context of patient care.

We organized the components of physicianship into separate domains that we call "the integrative disciplines," a term that requires some definition. *Integrative* refers to the unifying process that brings together knowledge and skills that otherwise remain apart. A physician can observe that a patient is in congestive heart failure *and* that she is poor. The integrative process sews together these two observations and forms a tapestry of limited access, unaffordable medication, or improper nutrition. *Discipline* refers to a branch of knowledge or teaching and to the competencies that follow when the discipline has been internalized. These competencies are more than attitudes: They are real; they can be observed; and they make a difference.

All told, this sourcebook describes the content of twenty integrative disciplines that collectively constitute a challenge to program directors and curriculum committees. The integrative disciplines, however, lie at the core of internal medicine and, in many ways, are the essence of the profession. To assist program directors and committees in developing educational approaches to these integrative disciplines, we arranged them in three tiers and presented them in the following order. First, are the *core values of internal medicine*: humanism, professionalism, and medical ethics. Residents will learn these disciplines largely through discussion, problem-solving exercises, workshops, and practical experience. Program leaders should not assume that residents are competent in these areas. Next, are the *characteristics, or salient expressions,* of these core values. This second tier of integrative disciplines includes lifelong learning, continuity of care, clinical method, interviewing, physical diagnosis, clinical epidemiology and quantitative reasoning, scientific literacy, legal medicine, management of quality of care, nutrition, and preventive medicine. These areas have their own vocabularies, operations, and concepts. They are likely to require at least some formal instruction in addition to opportunities for practice and formal feedback. The final tier comprises *integrative skills, or applications*, of the values and characteristics. This tier includes care delivered in specific settings and requires specific skill sets. Home care, nursing home care, occupational and environmental medicine, physical medicine and rehabilitation, practice management, and medical informatics all fit in this category. For these areas, theory may be less important than practice, and the principal learning technique is acquiring experience in realistic settings.

Inculcating the Essential Characteristics of the Internist

Educating residents in these integrative disciplines is akin to teaching the art of one's discipline. Learning these skills and attitudes is complex and absorbing, intuitive and creative . . . and it is possible. Learners acquire the characteristics of physicianship through several channels: Seminars provide abstract concepts; role models provide learning by example; and patients provide experiential learning.

Seminars

Seminars provide opportunities to focus on the core behaviors of internal medicine, including its values, attitudes, and behaviors. Seminars can include didactic information, exploration of personal experiences using critical incidents or similar techniques, and discussion. Many programs have had great success with seminars or group discussions organized around the integrative disciplines of humanism, professionalism, the clinical and practice method, management skills, and lifelong learning. Additional information about didactic methods in these areas appears in Chapter 8.

Role Modeling

Residents learn the characteristics of the internist from faculty who themselves manifest the highest standards of the profession. For a role model to be effective, however, he or she must take advantage of "teachable moments." Residents can learn the subtleties of clinical practice especially well when an expert steps back from a virtuoso performance, pauses to reflect out loud, and describes the ingredients of excellence. These reflections are also opportunities to address the value-laden aspects of medical care, by sharing with residents the personal sense of sacrifice and enrichment that professional behaviors entail.

Learning with Patients

In the clinics and on the wards, residents learn how to establish doctor-patient relationships that express the values of the profession. They learn to deal with simple and complex patients and with uncertainty. The partnership between physician and patient empowers both to engage in healing behaviors. Residents learn to recognize what they do not know and when to refer. They practice as members of a team and witness the benefits of effective team care. The closer the relationship between resident and patient, the more the resident learns. The intensity of the ward service and the continuity of the ambulatory setting complement one another; in each setting, residents learn something different about the characteristics of their profession.

A User's Guide to the Integrative Disciplines

The competencies suggested for each integrative discipline provide program directors with a resource, or checklist, that has been reviewed and endorsed by national panels of experts. These lists should prove useful as curriculum committees in individual programs decide how these important subjects will be learned. Beyond providing competency lists for the integrative disciplines, the Task Force hopes to be helpful here in two other ways. First, we suggest some of the likely venues and clinical rotations that exemplify how the most important of the integrative discipline competencies are used in clinical practice. Second, we provide a series of grids that curriculum committees can use to ensure that each competency finds its way into their program.

The grids display the competencies alongside two columns. The columns provide program directors and curriculum committees with a process to distribute competencies to specific clinical rotations if, in fact, that rotation is likely to provide opportunities for residents to become proficient in that competency. Alternatively, the program director and committee may decide that a particular competency warrants a more directive learning experience, such as a conference or seminar. For example, program directors can reasonably assume that residents will develop the competency, "Create and sustain doctor-patient relationships that maximize the likelihood of the best possible outcomes for the patients and the greatest personal satisfaction for the physician" in the context of their continuity practice. However, the competency, "Demonstrate skill in active listening, empathy, appropriate self-disclosure, empowering the patient, and stimulating the patient's growth and development" may require a workshop devoted to interviewing. If so, the program director would write "interviewing workshop" in the appropriate space on the grid. The list of competencies assigned to any specific workshop, seminar, or conference would then constitute the objectives of that particular learning program.

A final word on overlap and redundancy. Consistent with the approach taken to the clinical competency lists, the Task Force has eliminated excessive redundancy, as might be found, for example, in the overlapping disciplines of geriatrics and nursing home care or clinical epidemiology and prevention. Therefore, a competency that could reasonably appear on several lists may appear only once. The presence of a competency on one list or the other does not necessarily imply anything about the breadth or narrowness of any particular discipline. It may simply reflect a convenience for curriculum planning. Whenever possible, we cross-reference competencies that could equally well appear on another list ("see also").

THE INTEGRATIVE DISCIPLINES

FIRST TIER

Core Values of Internal Medicine

- Humanism

- Professionalism

- Medical Ethics

Humanism

Humanism in internal medicine should signify no vague exhortation to goodness but rather a set of defined knowledge, skills, and attitudes that brings about an admirable clinical process and desired health outcomes. Within the broad topic of humanism reside several core topics. This curriculum treats some of these, such as the medical interview, behavioral medicine, and medical ethics, as separate integrative disciplines, although they overlap with each other and with humanism as a discipline. Here we define other competencies that are not readily assigned to these related areas. Together these competencies embody the actual knowledge and skills underlying and essential to working with patients (and colleagues). They enable patients and physicians to deal with real problems, the full range of reactions and needs associated with medical problems and processes, and the life and lifestyle issues that contribute to health and disease.

See also: Medical Interview, Professionalism, Ethics, Continuity of Care, Nursing Home Care, and other clinical disciplines.

Competencies for the Humanistic Practice of Medicine

Competency	Learn in a seminar or conference (specify)	Learn as part of a clinical rotation (specify)
Create and sustain doctor-patient relationships that maximize the likelihood of the best outcome for the patients and the greatest personal satisfaction for the physician		
Be able to identify types of patient-physician relationships, factors promoting their relationships, and one's own relating style, preferences, and limitations		
In dealing with dying patients, demonstrate knowledge and skill in obtaining and interpreting advance directives for care at the end of life, and in providing comfort care, including managing the patient's pain and anxiety and the family's grief		
Recognize and appropriately manage so-called "difficult patients," including their personality disorders and problematic behavioral patterns		
Understand one's own personal reactions to difficult situations; use these reactions to generate explanatory hypotheses and to understand potential barriers to communication		
Understand the concept of the health belief model; know how to elicit it and how to work constructively in a patient-centered way with persons from different cultural groups		

Illustrative Clinical Experiences: Continuity clinic, oncology, geriatrics, nursing home rotations, psychiatry, and any clinical rotation that underscores the importance of humanism in medical practice.

Professionalism

Professionalism in medicine requires the physician to place the interest of the patient above the physician's self-interest. Professionalism aspires to altruism, accountability, excellence, duty, service, honor, integrity, and respect for others.

A physician's sense of self as a professional is under constant challenge and may require repeated, active reaffirmation to remain intact. Internal medicine's practitioners and teachers operate under ever-increasing imperatives for fast-paced, economically driven medical care. They no longer can assume that the circumstances of their practice will enhance their efforts to express the values of their profession in their work. Teachers cannot assume that their trainees will see these values in action. Quite the contrary, trainees may witness—and adopt—a standard of practice that is not consistently professional, unless their teachers and role models look inward and rediscover the ethical roots through which medicine has sustained its character as a profession. At risk in these daily brushes with subprofessional attitudes and behaviors are internal medicine's standards of excellence in patient care, education, and research.

Professionalism is a core set of values, attitudes, and behaviors that motivate physicians to make the interests of patients and society their first priority. The elements of professionalism, which have been identified by the American Board of Internal Medicine, from which this list is drawn, encompass 1) a commitment to the highest standards of excellence in the practice of medicine and in generating and disseminating knowledge; 2) a commitment to seek to know the interests of individual patients and to protect their interests; and 3) a commitment to be responsive to the health needs of society. These elements require residents to acquire the competencies that are listed below.

See also: Humanism, Legal Medicine, Ethics, Lifelong Learning, Medical Interviewing.

Competencies for Professionalism

Competency	Learn in a seminar or conference (specify)	Learn as part of a clinical rotation (specify)
Demonstrate a personal sense of altruism by consistently acting in one's patients' best interest		
Maintain accountability—to the patient, to society, and to the profession—by fulfilling all agreements, both written and implied		
Show a commitment to standards for lifelong excellence by continuously adding to one's knowledge of medicine and by drawing the distinction between knowledge that is based on high-quality evidence and knowledge from anecdote and personal experience		
Demonstrate a sustained commitment to service by accepting inconvenience to meet patients' needs, advocating for the best possible care for every patient, seeking active roles in professional organizations, and volunteering one's skills and expertise to advance the welfare of patients and the community		
Demonstrate honesty and integrity through one's behaviors by recognizing and avoiding conflicts of interest and relationships and by refusing to allow personal gain to supersede the best interest of patients		
Behave with high regard and respect for colleagues, other members of the health care team, and patients and their families		

Illustrative Clinical Experiences: All clinical rotations, but particularly those that exemplify clinicians' values and belief systems, such as continuity and community-based practice, free clinics and shelters, and venues in which the acuity of illness is high, such as intensive care units.

Medical Ethics

Ethics is the systematic application of values. Medical ethics focuses on the prevention, recognition, clarification, and resolution of ethics issues and conflicts that arise in the care of particular patients, and on the prevention and resolution of conflicts associated with ethical issues. Topics in clinical medical ethics include professional responsibility, informed consent, determination of decision-making capacity, truth-telling, confidentiality, and the physician's role in cost containment. Clinical medical ethics encompasses more than ethical quandaries and dilemmas; medical ethics also emphasizes the basic values that underlie clinical interactions, such as honesty, integrity, the primacy of the commitment to the patient's well-being, and compassion.

The general internist must be able to recognize ethical issues in clinical practice and identify hidden values and unacknowledged conflicts. Physicians must understand how common religious, cultural, and ethical beliefs affect patient preferences. Physicians also should demonstrate specific cognitive and behavioral skills, including basic knowledge of ethical and legal concepts; critical thinking about ethical issues; the capacity to justify a course of action; and the capacity to implement ethical decisions. Although general internists can handle most ethical issues, they should know when and how to seek the advice of an ethics consultant or committee.

See also: Legal Medicine, Humanism, Medical Interview, Professionalism, Critical Care, Geriatrics, Nursing Home, Oncology, Continuity Practice.

Competencies for Medical Ethics

Competency	Learn in a seminar or conference (specify)	Learn as part of a clinical rotation (specify)
Know how to inform patients and obtain voluntary consent for the general plan of medical care and specific diagnostic and therapeutic interventions		
Know what to do when the patient refuses a recommended medical intervention in both emergency and non-emergency situations		
Know what to do when a patient requests ineffective or harmful treatment		
Be able to assess a patient's decision-making capacity		
Know how to select the appropriate surrogate decision maker when the patient lacks decision-making capacity		
Understand the grounds on which surrogates should make decisions for patients who lack decision-making capacity		
Know the principles that apply when the physician must decide for a patient when the patient lacks decision-making capacity and there is no appropriate surrogate decision maker		
Be adept at broaching the subject of a dying patient's eventual death and discussing with the patient the extent of medical interventions at the end of life (see advance directives, below)		
Know how to handle the following situations related to end-of-life care		
• Withholding or withdrawing life-sustaining treatment, including nutrition and hydration		
• Communicating "bad news" and listening for the patient's and family's concerns		
• Writing "do not resuscitate" orders		
• Requests for physician-assisted suicide or euthanasia		
• Know how to address requests to breach confidentiality		
• Know the principle of truth-telling and how to implement it in situations involving information disclosure and medical errors		

Competencies for Medical Ethics (continued)

Competency	Learn in a seminar or conference (specify)	Learn as part of a clinical rotation (specify)
Understand the following ethical principles that underlie the fiduciary relationship with one's patients		
• Balancing obligations to patients with one's self-interest		
• Balancing obligations to patients with societal interests (for example, bedside rationing and case management)		
Know how to deal with the following forms of potential conflict of interest		
• Induced demand (physicians' ability to create a demand for their service)		
• Accepting gratuities from manufacturers		
Know the physician's obligation when he or she suspects that another health care provider is abusing alcohol or drugs or is professionally incompetent		
Know how to recognize and resolve ethical issues that arise in clinical research		

Illustrative Clinical Settings: Intensive care units, nursing homes, geriatrics units, oncology units, and anywhere that the values of the profession are discussed around realistic clinical situations.

THE INTEGRATIVE DISCIPLINES

SECOND TIER

Characteristics and Salient Expression of Internal Medicine's Core Values

- Lifelong Learning

- Clinical Method

- Continuity of Care

- The Medical Interview or History

- Physical Diagnosis

- Clinical Epidemiology and Quantitative Clinical Reasoning

- Clinical Pharmacology

- Scientific Literacy

- Legal Medicine

- Management of Quality of Health Care

- Nutrition

- Preventive Medicine

Lifelong Learning

Internists should be lifelong learners. They should be willing to adjust their concepts and practices in response to new evidence, to learn from their own experience and mistakes, and to improve the practice of medicine through quality improvement, innovation, and discovery.

Few attitudes are as important to the individual practitioner as the desire to learn. Internists must be able to assess their own learning needs and identify their own learning style. They must be aware of the gaps between the ideal, their own goals, and their actual performances. Never are these attitudes tested more severely than when the internist must come to terms with a mistake. Although painful to confront, errors are priceless opportunities for learning and self-improvement.

Although lifelong learning is an attitude, it is also a skill. Each internist should have a personal method for "keeping up." The options now include electronic databases as well as the more traditional approaches of regular reading, conference attendance, and discussion with consultants. Future internists may become members of "learning teams." These teams will use the techniques of quality improvement and learn from each other as they strive to improve individual and collective practices.

See also: Medical Informatics, Management of Quality, Clinical Epidemiology, Professionalism.

Competencies for Lifelong Learning

Competency	Learn in a seminar or conference (specify)	Learn as part of a clinical rotation (specify)
Develop a personal method for "keeping up" with new advances and changes in knowledge		
Participate actively in didactic programs and other learning experiences organized within a residency program		
Maintain an attitude of healthy skepticism and curiosity, as evidenced by thoughtful questioning, independent study, and critical analysis of published materials		
Demonstrate facility in using electronic databases, literature retrieval services, and computer-based diagnostic reasoning programs		
Be able to critically appraise the medical literature, identifying the strengths and weaknesses of an article and its relevance to one's patient population		
Acquire teaching skills in the ambulatory and inpatient settings		

Illustrative Clinical Settings: Any clinical setting in which residents are challenged to learn, but particularly continuity and inpatient rotations that imbue an attitude of rigor and evidenced-based practice.

The Clinical Method

Internists' clinical methods define the discipline of internal medicine as fully as do the age of patients in an internal medicine practice, the locations of care, and even the illnesses of adults. Concepts and understanding of disease, the location of care, and treatments change with time. But the methods used by internists—the essence of internal medicine—do not change. The clinical method is iterative, and each part informs the others. The clinical method encompasses the principles and practices used to solve an individual patient's problem through the interview and examination and by diagnosis, treatment, and observation. The process begins as the patient enters the examining room. The physician begins by asking the patient about the reason for the visit. The physician negotiates the activities for the visit and actively listens, all the while helping the patient tell of the story of the illness. The clinical method continues through the entire encounter and sustains the physician-patient relationship continuously and comprehensively.

See also: Medical Management, Continuity Care, Humanism, Clinical Epidemiology, Preventive Medicine, Medical Interviewing, Physical Examination, and Lifelong Learning.

Competencies for the Clinical Method

Competency	Learn in a seminar or conference (specify)	Learn as part of a clinical rotation (specify)
Demonstrate skill in generating hypotheses early in the interview by integrating the patient's demographic characteristics, the initial complaint, his or her appearance, and other information into a preliminary diagnostic opinion		
Obtain appropriate data from the interview, physical examination, and diagnostic tests to support or refute the leading hypotheses		
Accurately scan for asymptomatic diseases and their risk factors, applying evidence-based preventive health guidelines to the patient's population, preferences, and personal agenda		
Demonstrate diagnostic strategies that deal with ambiguous or incomplete data by the application of probabilistic reasoning, all the while being aware of not-to-be-missed diagnoses		
Utilize the literature, expert opinion, and colleagues to support one's diagnostic process		
Function as a personal health manager to organize, arrange, and monitor effective delivery of health services, particularly when patients have chronic or complicated illness		
Maintain accurate records, communicate effectively with other providers, and bridge the gaps that can occur when the focus of care shifts between office, hospital, home, or chronic care facility		

Illustrative Clinical Experiences: Any clinical setting that affords responsibility for patient care, particularly if role-model clinicians are present.

Continuity of Care

Continuity of care, along with comprehensive care and coordinated care, defines the general internist's practice. Although the outpatient office is the principal setting for the practice of general internal medicine, the hospital inpatient unit and even the intensive care unit are also important parts of the general internists' world. An appreciation of the importance of the physician-patient relationship, patient advocacy, case management, professionalism, and continuity should permeate all of these settings.

Some of the specific competencies of continuity of care overlap competencies found in other lists. Certainly, the clinical issues that form the substrate for continuity practice appear elsewhere. The purpose of this list is to identify the range of knowledge, skills, and attitudes that make the difference between episodic, fragmented, and occasionally ineffective care and the kind of care that is emblematic of the best that general internal medicine practice can provide.

See also: Professionalism, Ethics, Medical Management, Preventive Medicine, Clinical Epidemiology, History Taking, Clinical Method, and the clinical disciplines that compose outpatient practice.

Competencies for Continuity of Care

Competency	Learn in a seminar or conference (specify)	Learn as part of a clinical rotation (specify)
Be able to diagnose and manage the common clinical presentations of office-based adult medicine, including abdominal pain, change in mental status, dizziness, dyspnea, dysuria, fatigue, fever, headache, insomnia, pain syndromes, swelling, syncope and lightheadedness, upper respiratory infections, weight gain, and weight loss		
Demonstrate expertise in the frequently required office-based procedures, such as arthrocentesis, cerumen removal, diaphragm fitting, flexible sigmoidoscopy, incision and drainage of abscesses, splinting and bracing, and general wound care		
Know how to modify risk factors for disease by counseling to achieve behavioral change		
Collaborate effectively with members of the health care team and other health professionals		
Be able to use standard functional assessment questionnaires		
Maintain accurate and complete patient records		
Effectively use office-based triage systems and telephone-based care		
Practice efficiently so that patient care proceeds at an acceptable rate, appropriate for the nature of each encounter		

Illustrative Clinical Settings: Continuity practice in a hospital-based or community site.

The Medical Interview or History

Expertise in communication forms the core of an internist's set of skills and certainly is no less important than knowledge of disease. Internists should be masters of the medical interview. Following the seminal work of the Task Force on the Medical Interview (since renamed the Academy for the Doctor-Patient Relationship), the medical interview has been defined as the entire medium of physician-patient interaction. Many of the topics in this curriculum address this interaction. The clinical competencies cannot be acquired without disease-specific interview skills; likewise the population-based competencies depend directly on contextual knowledge and the ability to take a history appropriate for distinct settings and populations. Here we focus on the generic skills of interviewing. The competencies of the medical interview define what internists should know and be able to do in the discipline of medical interviewing (or history taking), as they communicate with, care for, and provide comfort to their patients.

See also: Humanism, Clinical Method, Continuity of Care, Psychiatry, and several of the clinical disciplines.

Competencies for the Medical Interview

Competency	Learn in a seminar or conference (specify)	Learn as part of a clinical rotation (specify)
Understand that the medical history has several stages—the opening, the characterization of symptoms and life setting, the review of symptoms, and the closing: each requires mastery		
Understand the interview's several functions: eliciting the data, pointing toward a diagnosis, forging a relationship, and healing		
Shape the interview to fit the individual characteristics of the patient and the patient's illness or symptoms		
Elicit the patient's history (story) and the context (family, occupational and social milieu) in which the illness or symptoms occur		
Be alert to the patient's verbal and nonverbal behaviors, which are often the way to obtaining the clearest, most consistent narrative of the illness or symptoms		
Develop verbal and nonverbal communication skills in order to facilitate communication, elicit the emotional content of the interview, and provide comfort		
Overcome barriers to communication, including those derived from cultural differences or physical and mental impairment		
Use the interview to identify cognitive impairment, anxiety, denial, and defensiveness; be able to manage each during the interview		
Take a history of sensitive topics, such as alcoholism, substance abuse, and sexual functioning and sexuality		
Engage the patient as an ally in treatment planning		

Illustrative Clinical Settings: Any setting that affords opportunities for reflection on communication skills and interviewing.

Physical Diagnosis

Even in this era of burgeoning diagnostic technology, the physical examination remains among the internist's most accurate set of tools. These skills play an essential role in estimating the pretest probability of disease, which is the starting point for test interpretation. Moreover, there is an increasing body of knowledge about accuracy of physical signs. In many instances, bedside assessment is superior to noninvasive technology; in almost all cases, it is more accessible and cost-effective. Expertise in physical diagnosis is a valued characteristic of the well-trained internist. Instruction in and evaluation of physical diagnosis skill should be part of every residency program's curriculum.

We present first a list of general competency objectives for physical diagnosis, followed by an organ-specific list of the physical findings and maneuvers with which all residents should be familiar.

See also: Clinical Method and the clinical competencies.

Competencies for Physical Diagnosis

Competency	Learn in a seminar or conference (specify)	Learn as part of a clinical rotation (specify)
Understand how to apply the concept of operating characteristics (specificity, sensitivity, and likelihood ratios) to the interpretation of physical examination findings		
Understand the pathophysiologic explanation for common physical findings		
Know when to *abandon* a physical finding because new evidence has impugned its validity and when to *adopt* new findings that have been shown to be clinically useful		
Examine patients efficiently and systematically, maximizing accuracy and completeness, ensuring that the patient is comfortable, and protecting the patient's modesty		
Use the physical examination in the context of the entire clinical database to evaluate the patient efficiently and effectively		
Know the content of the screening physical examination that is appropriate for each patient's age, sex, and particular risk factors		
Utilize repeated, focused physical examinations to follow the course of a patient's illness		
Use physical findings to make decisions in settings that do not allow for extensive diagnostic testing		

Illustrative Clinical Settings: Any clinical setting where physical diagnosis skills can be emphasized and reviewed.

Specific Physical Examination Findings

Cardiologic Physical Examination Findings

Blood Pressure

1. Measure blood pressure in the upper extremities (right and left arm)
2. Measure blood pressure in the lower extremities (in hypertensive patients)
3. Pulsus paradoxus
4. Tilt test (orthostatic change in heart rate and blood pressure)

Pulses

5. Carotid bruits and thrills
6. Irregularity of arterial pulse
7. Water hammer (Corrigan) pulse
8. Pulses parvus and tardus
9. Pulse deficit (in atrial fibrillation)

Neck Veins

10. Estimation of central venous pressure by inspection of the neck
11. Kussmaul's sign
12. Hepatojugular reflex
13. Cannon *a* waves
14. Pulsatile liver of tricuspid regurgitation
15. Giant *v* waves

Inspection and Palpation

16. Inspect the precordium for cardiac impulses
17. Detection of cardiac enlargement by percussion
18. Palpation for size and characteristics of the apex impulse
19. Right ventricular heave
20. Palpation for aortic stenosis thrill

Heart Sounds

21. Increased, decreased, or variability of S_1, S_2
22. Normal and abnormal splitting of S_2
23. S_3 gallop
24. S_4 gallop
25. Pericardial friction rub

Clicks

26. Mitral valve click
27. Ejection click
28. Presystolic click

Systolic Murmurs

29. Tricuspid regurgitation
30. Rivera-Carvallo's maneuver (accentuation of pulmonic and tricuspid valve murmurs)
31. Mitral insufficiency
32. Pulmonic stenosis
33. Ventricular septal defect
34. Aortic stenosis

Diastolic Murmurs

35. Mitral stenosis
36. Pulmonary regurgitation
37. Aortic regurgitation

Maneuvers

38. Hand-gripping maneuver (effect on murmurs)
39. Squatting maneuver (effect on murmurs)
40. Valsalva maneuver (effect on murmurs)

Pulmonary Physical Examination Findings

Breath Sounds

1. Bronchial breath sounds
2. Crackles (including distinguishing early from late sounds)
3. Vesicular breath sounds
4. Wheezing
5. Stridor
6. Late inspiratory squeak
7. Amphoric breath sounds

Palpation and Percussion

8. Abnormal tactile fremitus
9. Assessment of diaphragmatic excursion
10. Deviated trachea

Respiratory Patterns and Inspection

11. Paradoxical respiration
12. Respiratory alternans
13. Use of accessory muscles
14. Cheyne-Stokes respiration
15. Kussmaul's respiration

Additional Thoracic Findings and Maneuvers

16. Pleural friction rub
17. E to A egophony
18. Whispered pectoriloquy

Extra-thoracic Findings

19. Clubbing
20. Central cyanosis and acrocyanosis
21. Plethora of erythrocythemia
22. Edema, right ventricular heave, and other findings of cor pulmonale

Gastroenterologic/Abdominal Physical Examination Findings

Intestinal Signs

1. Changes in bowel sounds
2. Abdominal distention
3. Visible peristalsis
4. Succussion splash

Peritoneal Signs

5. Rebound tenderness
6. Iliopsoas sign

Abdominal Aortic and Vascular Signs

7. Abdominal aneurysm
8. Abdominal arterial murmurs and bruits

Liver, Spleen, and Portal Hypertension

9. Identify and palpate lower liver edge
10. Assess for splenic dullness at Traube's space
11. Percuss liver span
12. Palpate lower spleen edge
13. Fluid wave of ascites
14. Shifting dullness
15. Icterus
16. Skin findings of liver disease

Biliary Tract

17. Palpate enlarged gall bladder (Courvoisier's signal)
18. Murphy's sign

Additional Findings

19. Inguinal and scrotal hernias
20. Anal sphincter tone
21. Rectal masses

Ophthalmologic Physical Examination Findings

Inspection

1. Redness consistent with conjunctivitis, episcleritis, and iritis
2. Scleral icterus
3. Hordeolum, chalazion
4. Ptosis and dysconjugate gaze (myasthenia) of neuromuscular disorders
5. Blepharitis
6. Conjunctival petechiae

Pupillary Findings

7. Anisocoria
8. Afferent defect (Marcus-Gunn pupil)

Funduscopic Findings

9. Cataracts
10. Retinal exudates and hemorrhages
11. Blood or pus in anterior chamber
12. Proliferative and background diabetic retinopathy
13. Hypertensive and atherosclerotic retinopathy
14. Drusen (signs of macular degenerations)
15. Papilledema
16. Hollenhorst plaque (microembolic disease)

Test of Vision

17. Visual acuity
18. Test of visual fields

Otolaryngologic Physical Examination Findings

Ears

1. Findings of otitis externa
2. Findings of otitis media
3. Tympanic perforation
4. Hearing deficits

Nose and Sinuses

5. Palpate and percussion for sinus tenderness
6. Abnormalities of nasal mucosa
7. Nasal polyps
8. Nasal septal perforation

Oral Cavity and Tongue

9. Whitish plaques of candida infection
10. Leukoplakia and mucosal abnormalities suggesting malignancy (inspection and palpation)

11. Ulceration
12. Gingival hyperplasia
13. Gingivitis
14. Aphthous ulcers
15. Caries and periodontal disease
16. Atrophic glossitis
17. Macroglossia
18. Migratory glossitis

Oropharynx and Tonsils

19. Acute pharyngitis
20. Acute tonsillitis
21. Peritonsillar and abscess

Additional Findings

22. Salivary gland obstruction and/or infection
23. Salivary gland enlargement (including tumors)
24. Detection of cervical adenopathy
25. Palpation of thyroid
26. Nuchal rigidity
27. Findings of deep-tissue infection and cellulitis

Gynecologic and Genitourinary Physical Examination Findings

Breast

1. Breast mass
2. Breast discharge

Pelvic Examination Findings

3. Cervical tenderness
4. Vaginal discharge
5. Adnexal mass
6. Uterine enlargement and/or mass
7. Cervical mucosa abnormalities
8. Evidence of hypoestrogenism

Male Genitourinary Findings

9. Prostate enlargement
10. Prostate tenderness
11. Prostate mass
12. Testicular mass
13. Epididymal swelling and/or tenderness
14. Non-descended testicle
15. Signs of hypogonadism

Vascular/Extremities Physical Examination Findings

Circulation

1. Auscultation of carotid, femoral arteries
2. Palpation of carotid, femoral arteries
3. Palpation of peripheral pulses: popliteal, dorsalis pedis, posterior tibial, brachial, radial
4. Cyanosis
5. Changes in temperature
6. Edema
7. Clubbing
8. Palmar erythema
9. Splinter hemorrhages

Additional Findings

10. Dupuytren's contracture
11. Spooning of nails

Dermatologic Physical Examination Findings

(The findings are grouped for convenience; no classification scheme is implied.)

Inflammation and Infection

1. Open and closed comedones (acne)
2. Carbuncle and furuncle
3. Herpes simplex, zoster and varicella
4. Infestations (lice and scabies)
5. Tinea versicolor and corporis
6. Syphilis (primary and secondary)
7. Molluscum contagiosum
8. Acne rosacea
9. Verruca (warts)

Papulosquamous

10. Actinic keratosus
11. Eczema
12. Pityriasis rosea
13. Psoriasis
14. Seborrheic dermatitis
15. Lichen planus
16. Lichen simplex chronicum (neurodermatitis)

Skin Cancers and Related Disorders

17. Atypical nevus
18. Basal cell carcinoma
19. Malignant melanoma

20. Nevi
21. Squamous cell carcinoma
22. Angiomas

Allergic and Related Conditions

23. Contact dermatitis
24. Atopic dermatitis
25. Urticaria
26. Erythema multiforme/Stevens-Johnson syndrome

Vascular and Systemic

27. Erythema nodosum
28. Discoid lupus
29. Skin finding of systemic lupus erythematosus
30. Ischemic ulcer
31. Necrosis; gangrene
32. Livedo reticularis
33. Stasis ulcer and dermatitis
34. Petechiae/purpura/ecchymosis
35. Palpable purpura

Bullous Diseases

36. Pemphigus
37. Bullous pemphigoid

Additional Findings

38. Burns
39. Xerosis (dry skin)

Rheumatologic Physical Examination Findings

Temporomandibular

1. Findings of temporomandibular joint syndrome

Cervical Spine

2. Range of motion
3. Radiculopathy signs

Lumbosacral Spine

4. Range of motion
5. Localized tenderness
6. Radiculopathy signs (especially L4-5, L5-S1)
7. Sacroiliac tenderness
8. Inspect for kyphosis and abnormal lordosis

Shoulder

9. Range of motion
10. Palpation of biceps tendon groove
11. Palpation of subdeltoid bursa
12. Impingement syndrome findings
13. Opposed supination (biceps tendonitis)

Elbow

14. Range of motion
15. Swelling of olecranon bursitis
16. Tenderness in lateral epicondylitis
17. Ulnar nerve entrapment

Wrist and Hand

18. Swan neck deformity
19. Heberden's nodes
20. Bouchard's nodes
21. Carpal tunnel signs (Tinnels, Phelan's)
22. Thenar eminence atrophy

Hip

23. Range of motion (with pain referral patterns)
24. Asymmetry (including external rotation)
25. Tenderness of trochanteric bursitis

Knee

26. Range of motion and symmetry
27. Ballottment for fluid (and bulge sign)
28. Medial and collateral ligament tear signs
29. Anterior cruciate ligament tear (Lachman's maneuver)
30. Crepitation of osteoarthritis
31. Tenderness and swelling of prepatellar bursa
32. Tenderness over anserine bursa
33. Tibiopatellar tendinitis
34. Swelling of Baker's cyst
35. Signs of patellar femoral arthralgia (chondromalacia)

Ankle and Foot

36. Range of motion, tenderness and swelling
37. Ankle sprain
38. Tenderness of Achilles tendinitis
39. Signs of plantar fasciitis
40. Signs of podagra

Neurologic Physical Examination Findings

Higher-Level and Cortical Function

1. Mental status examination (including dementia and delusion)
2. Speech and language content
3. Asterixis

Movement, Gait, and Station

4. Parkinsonian tremor
5. Cogwheeling
6. Tardive dyskinesia
7. Ataxic or wide-based gait
8. Spastic gait
9. Parkinsonian gait
10. Intention (essential) tremor

Motor

11. Strength and symmetry of motor examination
12. Muscle tone (spasticity)
13. Pronator "drift"

Sensory

14. Abnormalities of pain (pinprick, light touch, position, vibration)
15. Romberg's sign

Cranial Nerves, Ocular and Oculomotor Function

16. Testing cranial nerves 2–10, 12
17. Oculomotor reflex (Doll's eyes)
18. Anisocoria
19. Pinpoint or dilated (unreactive) pupils
20. Horner's syndrome
21. Papilledema

Reflexes, Normal and Pathologic

22. Deep tendon reflexes
23. Babinski's sign
24. Hoffman's sign

Peripheral Nerves and Neuromuscular Findings (see also Musculoskeletal)

25. Fasciculations
26. Trousseau's sign
27. Chvostek's sign
28. Radial neuropathy
29. Median neuropathy
30. Ulnar neuropathy

Additional Findings

31. Cerebellar testing (upper and lower extremities)
32. Nuchal rigidity
33. Kernig's and Brudzinski's signs

Endocrinologic Physical Examination Findings

Pituitary

1. Growth retardation
2. Acromegaly
3. Galactorrhea

Thyroid

4. Goiter
5. Thyroid nodules
6. Exophthalmos
7. Findings of hyperthyroidism
8. Findings of hypothyroidism

Adrenal

9. Findings of hypoadrenocortisolism
10. Findings of hyperadrenocortisolism

Gonadal Disorders

11. Cryptorchidism
12. Klinefelter's syndrome habitus
13. Polycystic ovary disease findings
14. Findings of male hypogonadism
15. Findings of menopausal state

Bone Disorders

16. Paget's disease findings
17. Osteoporosis findings

Lipid Disorders

18. Skin and tender signs of hyperlipidemia

Diabetes

19. Neuropathy
20. Retinopathy

Clinical Epidemiology and Quantitative Clinical Reasoning

Clinical epidemiology is the study of how clinical questions (such as diagnosis, prognosis, and treatment) are answered by strong scientific research involving populations and groups of patients. Internists must find ways to cope with a rapidly changing evidence base for medicine, with clinical controversy, and with information overload. They should be able to assess the validity of published evidence for themselves. To do so requires understanding the basic clinical research strategies, such as study design, measurement, and analysis, and the meaning of terms used to describe research results in journals. Internists should also be able to judge the credibility of colleagues (authors of review articles, editorials, teachers, and consultants) who synthesize scientific evidence for them. Medical students do not necessarily acquire these abilities in medical school lectures or during teaching rounds; residency programs must teach this material, reinforce it by example, and monitor how well the housestaff use it in clinical care.

Dealing with uncertainty is one of the internist's fundamental skills. Quantitative clinical reasoning, also known as decision analysis, is the best method for using imperfect data to make decisions under conditions of uncertainty. Presented below are clinical epidemiology skills followed by skills of quantitative reasoning.

See also: Preventive Medicine, Informatics, Management of the Quality of Health Care.

Competencies for Clinical Epidemiology

Competency	Learn in a seminar or conference (specify)	Learn as part of a clinical rotation (specify)
Understand how bias and chance affect the accuracy of observations on individual patients		
Assess the validity of original research concerning diagnosis, prognosis, treatment, and prevention		
Know the strengths and weaknesses of randomized clinical trials, case-control studies, cohort studies (retrospective, prospective), and meta-analyses		
Demonstrate a practical strategy for judging the validity of colleagues' synthesis of clinical evidence (for example, review articles, continuing medical education courses, or consultant advice)		
Understand the meaning, uses, and limitations of statistical power, P values and confidence intervals, relative risk, attributable risk, and "number needed to treat"		

Competencies for Quantitative Clinical Reasoning

Competency	Learn in a seminar or conference (specify)	Learn as part of a clinical rotation (specify)
Understand how to estimate the pretest probability of a disease and how to use Bayes' theorem to estimate post-test probability		
Define and use sensitivity, specificity, and likelihood ratios of diagnostic information		
Know and be able to detect potential biases in estimates of sensitivity and specificity		
Understand the value of decision trees and expected value decision making		
Know how to measure patients' preferences		
Understand and utilize sensitivity analysis and cost-effectiveness analysis		

Illustrative Clinical Settings: Any clinical encounter is an occasion to learn these concepts. Settings particularly well suited are those that challenge residents to make evidenced-based decisions in areas of greater or lesser uncertainty and in settings where faculty exemplify and emphasize these concepts.

Clinical Pharmacology

Clinical pharmacology and therapeutics deals with the efficacy and safety of drugs, the optimal clinical use of drugs, and the development of new and improved drug therapies. It may draw on such disparate basic sciences as pharmacology, pharmacokinetics, pharmacodynamics, toxicology, and clinical trial design and analysis. Clinical activities emphasize consultation in therapeutic choice and monitoring and the evaluation of new therapies.

Competencies for Clinical Pharmacology

Competency	Learn in a seminar or conference (specify)	Learn as part of a clinical rotation (specify)
Know the basic pharmacokinetic parameters of drugs; apply this knowledge to drug monitoring and drug dosage regimen design and adjustment		
Describe a pharmacotherapeutic approach that includes definition of therapeutic objectives and options, selection of dose and parameters to monitor, and measurement of therapeutic outcome		
Be able to evaluate the individual patient's therapeutic response by monitoring drug levels, pharmacologic effects, and adverse reactions and by assessing individual variability in drug metabolism		
Know when to alter drug dosage because of altered drug disposition or conditions that place the patient at unusual risk		
Know the principles of adverse drug reactions, drug allergies, and drug interactions and how the characteristics of the patient may alter them		
Know how to use pharmacologic principles and information from poison control centers to diagnose and manage poisonings and drug overdose		
Understand national and local policies related to drug use, including • federal and state regulations • drug utilization review • ethical issues related to prescribing • experimental therapies • new drug development and FDA approval		

Illustrative Clinical Settings: Lectures, clinical electives, clinics, inpatient services.

Scientific Literacy

The basic science underlying normal human biology and disease is advancing rapidly. Moreover, practical application of new scientific knowledge to medical care seems to occur more and more quickly. These advances are exciting, but they are also challenging. General internists need to maintain their scientific literacy if they are to provide their patients with the best possible care. Residency training must play its role in supporting internists' need to maintain up-to-date knowledge of basic biomedical science.

The pace of scientific advance is so rapid that any list of topics with which residents should be conversant is likely to become obsolete quickly. Program directors should engage the faculty in deciding which topics to teach. Examples of current topics include cytokines, endothelial biology, cellular mechanisms of oncogenesis, and the biology of atherosclerosis. Lectures, seminars, and clinical rotations are venues in which to teach about basic biology and its expression in disease.

See also: Professionalism, Lifelong Learning, and several clinical disciplines.

Illustrative Clinical Settings: Any clinical rotation or elective is an opportunity to apply the principles of basic science to patient care.

Legal Medicine

Legal medicine, now often called health care law, has grown to become a legal specialty. In the United States, statute and common law, administrative regulation, and ethical constraints all constrain and regulate the practice of medicine. Legal medicine encompasses all of these topics. Some legal fundamentals, such as informed consent, advance directives, and confidentiality, affect clinical practice so often that internists should know how they may affect clinical practice. Other aspects of legal medicine either are encountered infrequently or are so complex that the prudent physician needs only to know when to seek legal counsel.

Medical schools do not teach these topics uniformly, and residency programs cannot assume that residents have a common knowledge base. Because the law varies from state to state, the curriculum will vary from program to program. Such common topics as malpractice and informed consent are obedient to national principles, yet their details are governed by state statutes and common law.

Residents acquire much of their understanding of legal medicine from discussions on rounds, during procedures, and while caring for ambulatory patients. Such informal teaching does not suffice for the core of health care law, which is a topic well-suited to didactic teaching. Traditional case-based teaching methods can then expand on this core material.

See also: Ethics, Management of Medical Practice, Clinical Method.

Competencies for Legal Medicine

Competency	Learn in a seminar or conference (specify)	Learn as part of a clinical rotation (specify)
Know the legal definition of privacy and its implications for medical care		
Discriminate correctly among requests to breach the confidentiality of patient records		
Identify patients who are incompetent to direct their own care and which of their surrogates are legally empowered to direct the patient's care		
Implement advance directives for end-of-life medical care		
Know the ethical and statutory constraints on the withdrawal or withholding of treatment		
Practice the methods of personal risk management (documentation, communication and instruction, informed consent, and follow-up) to avoid frivolous claims of malpractice		
Know statutory requirements to report events (for example, death, reportable diseases, abuse, and neglect) to civil authorities and know how to respond in order to ensure compliance with these regulations		
Know the administrative regulations that govern medical practice and know how to respond in order to be in compliance		
Know the principles of business law that affect the practice of medicine		
Know how bioethics and legal medicine relate to one another		

Illustrative Clinical Settings: Any clinical setting, but particularly those that involve conflicts that require the application of legal medicine principles for resolution.

The Management of the Quality of Health Care

In the past, efforts to exert control over the quality of health care have relied upon sanctioning of physicians after retrospective discovery of instances of poor quality care. The essence of the method was to find an error after it occurred and punish the person who made the error. This method has become outdated with the emergence of a new paradigm for quality management in industry in the United States and its application to health care. The new approach changes the production process so that the number of errors decreases. A motivation for applying this principle to health care is the emergence of managed care, with its focus on reducing costs while sustaining or improving the quality of care. The persuasiveness of current efforts to improve quality while reducing costs suggests that physicians-in-training will become involved in quality management and learn how to work with other professionals as members of quality management teams.

See also: Management of Medical Practice, Professionalism, Continuity of Care, Lifelong Learning, and Clinical Epidemiology.

Competencies for the Management of the Quality of Health Care

Competency	Learn in a seminar or conference (specify)	Learn as part of a clinical rotation (specify)
Be able to describe the training institution's quality management program		
Know methods for evaluating the effectiveness and efficiency of one's practice patterns		
Be able to describe how to use comparative data to measure variations in practice and thus identify best medical practices		
Know some of the standard measures of care (for example, functional status, return to work rates, measures of morbidity) and how to obtain them		
Know how to interpret the analytic tools utilized in quality improvement (for example, flow charts, fishbone diagrams, control charts)		
Be able to describe the methods used by external agencies and third-party payers to evaluate quality of care		
Know the principles underlying the study of practice patterns by using statistical profiling		
Be able to measure patient satisfaction in one's practice		
Know the methods used to develop practice guidelines and critical pathways and how physicians use them in the management of disease		
Be able to describe how to develop a quality improvement project		
Know the physician's role in efforts to improve health care		
Know how to lead a health care team that is trying to improve the quality of its services (understand team behavior, working with a team, and reshaping a team)		
Be able to describe measures of severity of illness and comorbidity		
Know the respective roles of the regulatory agencies involved in maintaining quality of medical care (for example, JCAHO, NCQA, HCFA, and state health care councils)		

Illustrative Clinical Settings: Although these competencies can be addressed in the context of clinical care, they are best acquired through participation in quality management teams and related activities.

Nutrition

Clinical nutrition focuses on the importance of nutrition in the maintenance of health and the interrelationship between nutrition and disease. Areas of interest for the general internist include enteral and parenteral nutritional support for hospitalized, homebound, or chronic care patients; nutritional support for surgical and trauma patients; and the role of nutrition in disease prevention. The curriculum should emphasize nutritional assessment and management of patients with nutritional deficiencies or excesses, hypersensitivities, eating disorders, nutritional diseases, and other pathologic conditions in which nutrition therapy would be beneficial.

See also: Geriatrics, Adolescent Medicine, Oncology, and several clinical disciplines.

Competencies for Nutrition

Competency	Learn in a seminar or conference (specify)	Learn as part of a clinical rotation (specify)
Identify from the history important risk factors for malnutrition, such as advanced age, poor detention, poverty and isolation, alcoholism, and chronic illness, particularly malignancy and gastrointestinal illness		
In a patient with risk factors for malnutrition or eating disorders, know how to screen for malnutrition through physical examination and appropriate procedures		
Review with a patient the dietary management for these common clinical conditions: obesity, hypertension, hyperlipidemia, diabetes, osteoporosis, congestive heart failure, and renal insufficiency		
Know the indications for and content of enteral and parenteral nutrition		

Illustrative Clinical Settings: Geriatrics, oncology unit, intensive care unit, adolescent unit, shelters, and other free-care clinics.

Preventive Medicine

Preventive medicine focuses on maintaining health and preventing disease, disability, and death. The basic components of preventive medicine include biostatistical principles and methodology; epidemiologic principles and methodology; planning, administration, and evaluation of health and medical programs; recognition and control of environmental and occupational hazards; social, cultural, and behavioral factors in medicine; and application of preventive principles and outcome measures in clinical practice. In the role of primary care physician, the general internist will engage in preventive medicine practice every working day. Mastery of this topic is essential and, importantly, a source of great satisfaction for general internists.

See also: Clinical Epidemiology, Continuity of Care, Clinical Method, Management of the Quality of Health Care.

Competencies for Preventive Medicine

Competency	Learn in a seminar or conference (specify)	Learn as part of a clinical rotation (specify)
Understand the principles of the determinants of the risk for disease		
Understand the principles of periodic health appraisal and the role of screening		
Understand the principles of age-specific profiles of risk		
Understand the principles of prophylaxis of disease		
Understand the principles of counseling to reduce risk		
Know the principles of investigating an epidemic		
Know the methods of behavior modification, risk assessment, and risk modification		
Know how to apply basic principles of critical evaluation of the literature to the study of screening and disease prevention		
Know the principles of office-based strategies for enhancing the delivery of preventive services		
Know the current adult preventive services recommendations of the U.S. Preventive Services Task Force, the American College of Physicians, or the Canadian Task Force on the Periodic Health Examination		

Illustrative Clinical Settings: Continuity practice, community-based practice.

THE INTEGRATIVE DISCIPLINES

THIRD TIER

Settings and Practices That Exemplify the Integrative Disciplines

- Home Care

- Nursing Home Care

- Occupational and Environmental Medicine

- Physical Medicine and Rehabilitation

- Management of Medical Practice

- Medical Informatics

Home Care

A consequence of the success of modern medicine is a proliferation of chronic disease and disability. Most people now face years of living with some progressive dependency and disability. Nursing-home beds already outnumber hospital beds, and for every person in a nursing home three more with similarly severe disabilities receive their care at home. Families alone, under their physician's guidance, provide 80% of the care for these homebound, frail patients. Younger patients, particularly those who are functioning well, also make increasing use of home services for infusion of medication, short-term recovery from injury, and other reversible situations.

To be effective in providing and supervising care for patients in their homes, a physician must build upon a mastery of traditional internal medicine by acquiring the following skills: 1) comprehensive advance planning; 2) assessment of the environment and the support system; 3) care oversight, team leadership, and standard setting; 4) compliance and confrontation with regulation; 5) financing of care over time; and 6) organization of services and continuous quality improvement. Also, the home setting is a particularly good setting in which to learn nutritional assessment, prevention and rehabilitation services, coordination of ancillary services, physical diagnosis, skin care of a bedridden patient, and care of the dying.

See also: Geriatrics, Nursing Home, Legal Medicine, and Management of Medical Quality.

Competencies for Home Care

Competency	Learn in a seminar or conference (specify)	Learn as part of a clinical rotation (specify)
Negotiate a plan of care that accounts for the wishes and preferences of the patient and family members		
When managing a patient at home, rely on basic clinical skills and avoid, as much as possible, unnecessary testing and hospitalization		
Be an effective supervisor of family caregivers and other health care providers		
Assess physical, psychological, and social function in the home		
Know the principles that guide successful implementation of multiple-drug regimens in the home setting, where many factors can interfere with compliance		
Distinguish between and know how to use the services provided by in-home therapies, respite services, day hospital or day care, visiting nurses, hospices, hospitals, consultant care providers, home health aides, and equipment suppliers		
Know the regulations and financing protocols that shape home care practice (Medicare, Medicaid, MediGap, and federal and state quality assurance and elder abuse regulations)		
Know the process for certifying that services are medically necessary		
Know the symptoms and signs that indicate that the patient is near death and know about strategies to alleviate suffering		
Know the administrative and legal arrangements when a patient dies outside of the hospital (pronouncing and certifying, communicating with the medical examiner and funeral director, and managing the dead body)		

Illustrative Clinical Settings: These competencies are best acquired in the management of patients in home settings as part of a block experience in home care. However, valuable experience in management of homebound patients also can be obtained during continuity practice experiences, inpatient medicine, nursing home, and geriatric rotations.

Nursing Home Care

Many adults face a long period of decline in the grip of chronic illness, such as Alzheimer's disease, or in the aftermath of an acute illness, such as a stroke. Many of these individuals will live out their days in a nursing home. Others will spend a short period in a nursing home as part of a successful convalescence after hospitalization. Physicians must be effective in the nursing home setting.

See also: Geriatrics, Home Care, Humanism, Medical Ethics, Legal Medicine, Nutrition, and several clinical disciplines

Competencies for Nursing Home Care

Competency	Learn in a seminar or conference (specify)	Learn as part of a clinical rotation (specify)
Know the special characteristics of history taking and physical examination in frail, disabled, elderly people		
Know the standardized instruments for assessing physical function, cognition, affect, and gait		
Be able to manage clinical conditions that are prevalent in nursing home patients, including infections, dementia, depression, urinary incontinence, falls, immobility, movement disorders, pressure sores, and polypharmacy		
Know regulations that apply to nursing home care (for example, use of physical restraints and psychotropic medications)		
Know the principles of rehabilitation in the nursing home and the concept of excess disability		
Know the levels of care that are considered appropriate for various types of facilities		
Know the role of the nursing home director		
Be able to describe the financing of long-term care		
Know how to function as part of an interdisciplinary nursing home team		
Be practiced in the telephone management of patient-care problems in the nursing home		
Be able to coordinate care between settings (acute care hospital, nursing home, home)		

Illustrative Clinical Settings: Nursing home and skilled-care facility rotations.

Occupational and Environmental Medicine

Occupational and environmental medicine is concerned with the diagnosis, treatment, and prevention of disease caused by agents in the environment. It focuses on preventing and treating occupational diseases and injuries; controlling or assessing health hazards in both the workplace and living environments; and fostering employee and public health through clinical care, education, and counseling programs. The specialty of occupational medicine requires a general health care orientation; the ability to provide clinical management in the work environment; the ability to work with both labor and management; and specific training in industrial hygiene, toxicology, biostatistics, and epidemiology. The general internist needs to know about health hazards in the home or workplace, how to do a preliminary evaluation, when to refer to an occupational medicine specialist, and how to assist in long-term management of work-related illness and disability.

See also: Legal Medicine, Clinical Epidemiology, Physical Medicine and Rehabilitation, Preventative Medicine Interviewing, and several clinical disciplines, including Pulmonary, Dermatology, and Musculoskeletal Medicine.

Competencies for Occupational and Environmental Medicine

Competency	Learn in a seminar or conference (specify)	Learn as part of a clinical rotation (specify)
Know how to take both a systematic occupational and environmental screening history and how to take an in-depth history when the patient's complaints or physical findings suggest an occupational or environmental health hazard		
Know the principles that help the physician decide whether an illness is caused by health hazards in the living and working environments		
Know how to apply epidemiologic principles to the evaluation of individual patients and, once a risk is identified, to coworkers and the community at large		
Be able to describe the basic principles of disease prevention and how to apply them to occupational and environmental effects on health		
Be able to counsel patients and others at risk about potential hazards in the community and workplace		
Know how to assess impairment and disability		
Be able to describe the physician's role in disability programs, including worker's compensation and Social Security		
Know how to evaluate complaints that could be environment-related and know when to refer to a specialist in occupational medicine		
Know the ethical, legal, and regulatory concerns specific to occupational and environmental medicine		

Illustrative Clinical Settings: Continuity practice, community-based practice, occupational health rotations.

Physical Medicine and Rehabilitation

The general internist will be responsible for care of many patients who may have suffered neuro-musculoskeletal system impairments that have resulted in residual disability. As a primary care provider, the general internist will need to be aware of the effects of such disabilities on other body systems and on the patient's ability to perform the routine activities of daily living and to fulfill various societal roles. The general internist will have the crucial role of ensuring continuity of care when the patient with multiple medical problems requires intervention from many health care professionals.

See also: Occupational Medicine, Musculoskeletal Medicine, Legal Medicine, Neurology, Geriatrics, and Nursing Home.

Competencies for Physical Medicine and Rehabilitation

Competency	Learn in a seminar or conference (specify)	Learn as part of a clinical rotation (specify)
Know the differences among impairment, disability, and handicap		
Know how to diagnose and manage the common musculoskeletal disorders, including fibromyalgia, myofascial pain, repetitive motion disorders, and overuse syndromes		
Know how to recognize the complications of prolonged bed rest (contractures, pressure sores, deep venous thrombosis, osteoporosis, muscular deconditioning, and others)		
Be able to describe various physical medicine treatment modalities, including diathermy, ultrasound, electrical stimulation, and others		
Know the physiologic effects of aerobic exercise		
Know the various types of therapeutic exercises		
Be able to describe the health care team for rehabilitative medicine and the roles of allied health professionals (for example, physical therapist, occupational therapist, psychologist, speech and language pathologist, prosthetist, orthotist, and others)		
Know when to use the various assistive devices that may reduce disability, including wheelchairs, prosthetics, orthotics, and others		
Know the principles of evaluation and management of chronic pain		
Know the methods for minimizing long-term disability from acute illnesses (for example, prophylaxis against venous thrombosis, bed sores, contractures)		
Be able to assess the effects of impairment on a patient's daily function		

Illustrative Clinical Settings: Nursing home, geriatric unit, rehabilitation center, neurology rotation, rheumatology rotation, cardiopulmonary rehabilitation unit.

The Management of Medical Practice

The principal focus of medical residency training is the prevention, diagnosis, and management of disease. A medical curriculum that focuses on these topics will prepare a resident to care for patients, but it will not fully prepare him or her to practice medicine. Medical practice occurs in a context that includes payment for medical services, an office and its staff, and systems to ensure that medical care in the practice never wavers from a high standard. All practicing physicians must understand this context in order to obtain the medical outcomes that they are capable of achieving.

Physicians need to understand the economic context of medical practice. Their needs will depend partly on the circumstances of practice. Physicians who work in small groups may negotiate directly over contracts with payers. Physicians in large groups that provide the administrative support for contracting will have different needs. The residency training program should provide an understanding of the economics of medical care sufficient to prepare for the varied circumstances of practice.

See also: Legal Medicine, Management of Quality.

Competencies for the Management of Medical Practice

Competency	Learn in a seminar or conference (specify)	Learn as part of a clinical rotation (specify)
Know the basic systems of payment for health care (indemnity plans, managed indemnity plans, capitation)		
Know how the forms of medical practice differ from one another (solo practice, group practice, preferred provider organizations, independent practice associations, vertical integration, networks, staff or group HMO)		
Know the principal types of payers for health care (Medicare; Medicaid; Blue Cross–Blue Shield; insurance companies, both for-profit and nonprofit; and the Department of Veterans Affairs)		
Understand the basic concepts of managing health care systems (utilization management, practice profiling, risk management, continuous quality improvement, managed care, measurement of outcomes, meeting national standards, federal laws affecting the organization of medical practice)		
Be prepared to negotiate effectively when deciding to take a job opportunity (salary and benefits, practice style, job description)		
Have a basic knowledge of basic business skills (accounting, personnel management, insurance billing, accounts receivable, collections, writing a job description, procedure and service coding, evaluating health plans, evaluating contracts)		

Illustrative Clinical Settings: Continuity practice sites, particularly if they expose residents to community practices, and inpatient rotations.

Medical Informatics

To provide efficient, effective patient care, internists must be highly proficient information managers. The volume and complexity of medical knowledge and data have outstripped the internist's ability to function optimally without support from information management tools. To make optimal use of the computer-based information resources that are available today requires an understanding of their strengths and limitations and of the issues involved in implementing them in clinical practice. Internal medicine residents should understand how to use current technologies and be able to adapt as new tools become available.

See also: Lifelong Learning, The Clinical Method, Continuity of Care, and Clinical Epidemiology.

Competencies for Medical Informatics

Competency	Learn in a seminar or conference (specify)	Learn as part of a clinical rotation (specify)
Know enough basic computer concepts and terminology to be well-informed in purchasing and using computers and peripheral devices, computer communication hardware, operating systems, general-purpose software, and important patient care–related clinical software		
Know essential aspects of file organization, hard- and floppy-disk information storage, protection from data loss, and basic issues related to computers and copyright law		
Be able to use basic word processing, spreadsheet, database, desktop publishing, and desktop presentation technology; know how to adapt these programs to medical uses		
Be able to identify, evaluate, select, and appropriately use electronic sources of medical knowledge, e.g., CD-ROMs, the Internet, decision support, and continuing medical education software, and literature searching programs		
Be able to identify, evaluate, select, and appropriately use computer systems for managing patient and practice information		
Be able to identify, evaluate, select, and appropriately use computer systems for educating patients		
Be able to identify, evaluate, select, and appropriately use portable computing devices to facilitate the mobile management of patient and practice data and medical knowledge		

Illustrative Clinical Settings: Anywhere that provides residents with the necessary equipment, instruction, and encouragement to apply these tools to actual clinical situations and needs.

CHAPTER 6

THE CLINICAL COMPETENCIES

This chapter contains the clinical presentations, procedure skills, tests, and clinical conditions in which internal medicine residents should attain competency by the end of graduate medical training. They are divided into lists that cover clinical organ and system-based disciplines, population-based disciplines, and site-specific disciplines (see Contents for a complete listing). We have gathered laboratory tests and procedures that are commonly done for diseases of many organ systems into a single list and present these first in order to obviate the need to repeat them for each discipline.

The format of the clinical competency lists follows a template developed by the FCIM Curriculum Task Force. Each list begins with an overview that briefly describes the scope of the discipline and the role of the general internist in that discipline. A list of common clinical presentations follows, including both symptoms and physical findings. Next, procedure skills specific to the discipline are listed. "Primary Interpretation of Tests" includes those tests that the resident should be able to do and "read" independently. For example, understanding the results of a laboratory study would not belong here, but ability to examine and interpret a Gram stain does belong. "Ordering and Understanding Tests" refers to tests that are ordered by laboratory and radiology requisition forms. The trainee is not expected to develop competence in actually doing these studies but should understand when to order them and the significance of their results.

The tables of "clinical conditions" list those conditions for which residents should obtain knowledge in diagnosis and management and understand when referral is indicated. The program director can characterize each condition by a priority rating of 1, 2, or 3 and then "assign" it to a learning venue. Through these priority scores, the Task Force sought to help program directors identify the most important and prevalent conditions and to decide how to apportion time between patient care experiences and didactic teaching in specific rotations. The Task Force used a consensus process to assign a priority score to each condition. A program director may adopt the Task Force's priority score for a competency or may substitute a rating that reflects local opinion and needs.

User's Guide to the Clinical Competency Lists

The best way to learn a competency is to take personal responsibility as principal caregiver for a patient with the clinical condition. Achieving this goal for each competency in the Task Force Report is not feasible in a 3-year curriculum.

Priorities, therefore, become important. The recommended priority score for each clinical competency represents a consensus of internists about the competency's importance and should guide program directors in making choices. Program directors can use the recommended priorities as a starting point for their local curriculum development process.

This priority scoring system requires several disclaimers. First, its purpose is to suggest preferred ways of learning, not to imply a hierarchy of expected levels of competence. We expect residents to strive for the same level of competence in a priority 1 competency as they do for a priority 3 competency. This disclaimer implies a second caveat: The priority scoring system does not imply that generalists are less competent to provide care for a disease with a lower priority score. Finally, just as the competencies themselves are not surrogates for requirements, neither should a high priority score imply a requirement. With this curriculum, internal medicine states its aspirations for excellence in residency education; it does not aim to establish minimum standards.

Priority 1: Because this condition is so important, the preferred way to learn about it is by taking personal responsibility for the care of patients with the condition (writing an initial evaluation and taking responsibility for ongoing care during an episode of illness; "direct patient care"; hands-on patient care). Priority 1 conditions are relatively frequent and important to learn. Housestaff should seek the opportunity to care for patients with this condition.

Priority 2: Because patients with this condition occur less frequently than patients with priority 1 conditions, it is not realistic to expect all housestaff to have principal responsibility for the care of patients who suffer from it. Nonetheless, exposure to the experience of patients with this condition is important for learning about it. Means to this end include a clinic-based discussion of a patient, seeing a patient in a group, and being a member of a team caring for the patient. Using a computer simulation of case management may suffice. As compared with priority 1 conditions, priority 2 conditions are less frequent but equally important to learn.

Priority 3: Residents can learn about this condition by reading or attending a lecture. As compared with priority 1 and priority 2 conditions, the condition occurs less frequently or is less important, or both. However, it should find a place in the curriculum, and it is more important than other clinical conditions that did not even "make the list."

The format of the "clinical conditions" section of each competency list integrates the list of competencies with the worksheet that the program director will use to assign each competency to a learning venue or rotation. The left-hand column contains the list of competencies. The next columns contain the Task Force's priority rating for the competency and a space to write in the program's priority rating. The next several columns correspond to the different learning venues (four columns for outpatient venues and one column for the inpatient venue). The right-hand column contains a space to describe any didactic teaching that will be used for learning that competency. In completing the grids, assigning competencies to rotations and identifying needed content for didactic programs, local curriculum committees will, in effect, be creating subject-specific mini-curricula that can be used to 1) determine the length of a given rotation in relationship to other rotations and 2) provide objectives that can guide learning, both clinical and didactic, at a given site.

Common Laboratory and Test Interpretation Skills*

Procedures

Be able to identify proper indications and safely perform:

- Lumbar puncture
- Flexible sigmoidoscopy
- Bladder catheterization
- Thoracentesis
- Paracentesis
- Gram stain of fluids and secretions
- Insertion of intravenous central catheters (peripheral and central)
- Arterial puncture

Primary Interpretation of Tests

Be able to inspect and interpret, or "read," data from:

- Chest x-ray
- Abdominal flat plate and upright x-ray
- Arterial blood gases
- Serum electrolytes and routine chemistry panel
- Liver function tests
- Coagulation studies
- Urine analysis
- Peripheral smear
- Electrocardiogram
- Office spirometry

*These are generic procedures and skills that several of the competency areas require. Listing them here obviates the need to list them repeatedly in the competency lists that follow.

THE CLINICAL COMPETENCIES

Organ and System Competencies

- Allergy and Immunology

- Cardiovascular Illness

- Dermatology

- Endocrinology and Metabolism

- Gastroenterology

- Hematology

- Infectious Disease

- Nephrology

- Neurology

- Oncology

- Ophthalmology

- Otolaryngology

- Psychiatry

- Pulmonary Medicine

- Rheumatology

Allergy and Immunology

Overview

Allergy and immunology involves the management of disorders related to hypersensitivity or altered reactivity caused by release of immunologic mediators or by activation of inflammatory mechanisms. An understanding of immunology is essential for mastery of subspecialty areas within all of the major disciplines of internal medicine and most of its allied specialties.

The general internist should be able to offer primary care for several diseases involving altered immunity or hypersensitivity. For these diseases, the general internist should be able to initiate diagnostic evaluation and therapy with or without the help of a subspecialist. The general internist should also be able to recognize many other diseases in which altered immunity plays an important role.

Common Clinical Presentations

- Anaphylaxis
- Conjunctival and bulbar inflammation, chemosis, ocular pruritus
- Dyspnea, cough, wheezing, sputum production, use of accessory muscles of respiration
- Nasal obstruction and pruritus, rhinorrhea, sneezing
- Skin whealing, angioedema, bullous formation, eczematous and papular eruptions, morbilliform rashes, purpura, pruritus

Procedure Skills

- Spirometry and spirometric response to bronchodilators
- Wright-Giemsa stain of nasal and pulmonary secretions

Primary Interpretation of Tests

- Delayed-hypersensitivity skin tests

Ordering and Understanding Tests

- Drug desensitization protocols
- Computed tomography of lungs, sinuses
- Immediate skin tests for IgE-mediated reactions to inhalants, food, certain drugs
- In vitro test for specific IgE
- Levels of complement components, C1 esterase inhibitor
- Methacholine inhalation challenge
- Patch tests
- Prick and intradermal skin tests
- Pulmonary function tests (including spirometry, lung volume, diffusion)
- Serum immunoglobulin levels
- Serum theophylline levels
- T- and B-cell quantitation and subtyping (CD classification)
- Total eosinophil count

In-depth knowledge of clinical conditions, including principles of management and indications for referral.

ALLERGY AND IMMUNOLOGY

Competency	Priority		Preferred Learning Venues					
			Outpatient			Other	Inpatient	Didactic
	FCIM Task Force	Residency Program	Continuity Clinic	Subspecialty Clinic	Other			
Allergic rhinitis/sinusitis	1							
Anaphylaxis	2							
Asthma	1							
Contact dermatitis	2							
Drug allergies	1							
Hypersensitivity pneumonias	2							
Hypersensitivity (small vessel) vasculitis	2							
Primary immunodeficiency	3							
Urticaria	1							

Key: 1 = direct patient responsibility preferred; 2 = any other form of learning that is centered on a patient; 3 = lectures/seminars/reading suffice.

Cardiovascular Illness

Overview

Cardiology is the prevention, diagnosis, and management of disorders of the cardiovascular system, including ischemic heart disease, cardiac dysrhythmias, cardiomyopathies, valvular heart disease, pericarditis and myocarditis, endocarditis, congenital heart disease in adults, hypertension, and disorders of the veins, arteries, and pulmonary circulation. Management of risk factors for disease and early diagnosis and intervention for established disease are important elements of cardiology.

The general internist should be able to provide primary and secondary preventive care and initially manage the full range of cardiovascular disorders. The need for additional competencies in cardiovascular disease will depend on the availability of a cardiologist in the primary practice setting. In some communities, the general internist may be responsible for management of more complex cardiovascular disorders that require intensive hemodynamic monitoring (for example, balloon-tipped pulmonary artery catheters) in the intensive care unit.

Common Clinical Presentations

- Abnormal heart sounds or murmurs
- Chest pain
- Dyspnea
- Effort intolerance, fatigue
- Hypertension
- Intermittent claudication
- Leg swelling
- Palpitations
- Peripheral vascular disease
- Risk factor modification
- Shock, cardiovascular collapse
- Syncope, lightheadedness

Procedure Skills

- Advanced cardiac life support
- Insertion of balloon-tipped pulmonary artery catheter (optional)
- Insertion of temporary pacemaker (optional)

Primary Interpretation of Tests

- Stress electrocardiography (optional)

Ordering and Understanding Tests
- Ambulatory electrocardiographic monitoring
- Echocardiography
- Electrophysiology testing
- Left ventricular catheterization and coronary angiography
- Nuclear scan wall motion study
- Right ventricular catheterization (including flotation catheter)
- Stress electrocardiography and thallium myocardial perfusion scan
- Tilt-table physiology study

In-depth knowledge of clinical conditions, including principles of management and indications for referral.

CARDIOVASCULAR ILLNESS

Competency	Priority		Preferred Learning Venues					
			Outpatient			Inpatient		Didactic
	FCIM Task Force	Residency Program	Continuity Clinic	Subspecialty Clinic	Other		Other	
Arrhythmias								
Atrial	1							
Conduction abnormalities	1							
Ventricular	1							
Pacemaker management	3							
Congenital heart disease	2							
Congestive heart failure								
Acute pulmonary edema	1							
Chronic congestive heart failure	1							
Coronary artery disease								
Angina pectoris, chronic stable	1							
Angina pectoris, unstable	1							
Myocardial infarction, complicated	1							
Myocardial infarction, uncomplicated	1							
Myocardial infarction follow-up	1							
Postoperative care (CABG, PTCA)	1							
Endocarditis	1							

CARDIOVASCULAR ILLNESS (CONT.)

Competency	Priority		Preferred Learning Venues					
	FCIM Task Force	Residency Program	Continuity Clinic	Outpatient Subspecialty Clinic	Outpatient Other	Other	Inpatient	Didactic
Hypertension								
Chronic stable hypertension	1							
Hypertensive crisis	1							
Secondary hypertension	1							
Myocardial disease								
Cardiomyopathy	2							
Myocarditis	2							
Pericardial disease								
Acute pericarditis	1							
Pericardial tamponade	2							
Preoperative evaluation of the cardiac patient	1							
Valvular heart disease	1							
Vascular disease								
Aortic disease	1							
Arterial insufficiency	1							
Chronic venous stasis	1							
Deep venous thrombosis	1							
Aneurysm (atherosclerotic, mycotic)	2							
Aortic dissection	2							

Key: 1=direct patient responsibility preferred; 2=any other form of learning that is centered on a patient; 3=lectures/seminars/reading suffice.

Dermatology

Overview

Dermatology is the management of disorders of the skin, mucous membranes, and adnexal structures, including inflammatory, infectious, neoplastic, metabolic, congenital, and structural disorders. Competence in medical and surgical interventions and dermatopathology are important facets.

The general internist should have a general knowledge of the major diseases and tumors of the skin. He or she should be proficient at examining the skin; describing findings; and recognizing skin signs of systemic diseases, normal findings (including benign growths of the skin), and common skin malignancies. The general internist should be able to diagnose and manage a variety of common skin conditions and make referrals where appropriate.

Common Clinical Presentations

- Abnormalities of pigmentation
- Eruptions (eczematous, follicular, papulosquamous, vascular, vesiculobullous)
- Hair loss
- Hirsutism
- Intertrigo
- Leg ulcer
- Mucous membrane ulceration
- Nail infections and deformities
- Pigmented lesion
- Pruritus
- Purpura
- Skin papule or nodule
- Verrucous lesion

Procedure Skills

- Application of chemical destructive agents for skin lesions, e.g., warts and molluscum, condyloma
- Incision, drainage, and aspiration of fluctuant lesions for diagnosis or therapy
- Scraping of skin (for potassium hydroxide, mite examination)
- Skin biopsy (punch)
- Cryotherapy

Primary Interpretation of Tests

- Microscopic examination for scabies, nits, etc.
- Tzanck smear

Ordering and Understanding Tests

- Dark-field microscopy
- Fungal culture
- Skin biopsy

In-depth knowledge of clinical conditions, including principles of management and indications for referral.

DERMATOLOGY

Competency	Priority		Preferred Learning Venues					
			Outpatient			Other	Inpatient	Didactic
	FCIM Task Force	Residency Program	Continuity Clinic	Subspecialty Clinic	Other			
Abscess	1							
Cellulitis	1							
Condyloma	1							
Cyst	1							
Eczematous reaction pattern								
Acute contact dermatitis	1							
Atopic dermatitis	1							
Stasis dermatitis	1							
Dyshidrotic eczema	2							
Nummular eczema	3							
Erythema nodosum	2							
Follicular disease								
Acne	1							
Rosacea	1							
Malignancy and premalignancy								
Actinic keratosis	1							
Basal cell carcinoma	2							
Melanoma	2							
Squamous cell carcinoma	2							
Molluscum contagiosum	2							

Key: 1 = direct patient responsibility preferred; 2 = any form of learning that is centered on a patient; 3 = lectures/seminars/reading suffice.

DERMATOLOGY (CONT.)

Competency	Priority		Preferred Learning Venues						
			Outpatient				Inpatient	Didactic	
	FCIM Task Force	Residency Program	Continuity Clinic	Subspecialty Clinic	Other	Other			
Papulosquamous reaction pattern									
Fungal, yeast infections	1								
Psoriasis	1								
Seborrheic dermatitis	1								
Lichen planus	2								
Syphilis	2								
Paronychia, folliculitis	1								
Pityriasis rosea	2								
Scabies	2								
Skin ulcers	1								
Skin signs of systemic disease									
Diabetes mellitus	1								
Liver disease	1								
Thrombocytopenia	1								
Kaposi's sarcoma	2								
Lupus erythematosus	2								
Sepsis	2								
Thyroid disease	2								
Dermatomyositis	3								
Gastrointestinal polyposis	3								
Inflammatory bowel disease	3								
Internal malignancy	3								
Rheumatoid arthritis	3								
Scleroderma	3								

DERMATOLOGY (CONT.)

Competency	Priority		Preferred Learning Venues					
			Outpatient			Other	Inpatient	Didactic
	FCIM Task Force	Residency Program	Continuity Clinic	Subspecialty Clinic	Other			
Vascular reaction pattern								
Drug hypersensitivity	1							
Urticaria	1							
Viral exanthems	1							
Erythema multiforme	2							
Toxic epidermal necrolysis	3							
Vasculitis	3							
Vesiculobullous reaction pattern								
Herpes simplex infection	1							
Herpes zoster infection	1							
Varicella	1							
Bullous pemphigoid	2							
Pemphigus vulgaris	2							
Warts	1							

Key: 1 = direct patient responsibility preferred; 2 = any form of learning that is centered on a patient; 3 = lectures/seminars/reading suffice.

Endocrinology, Diabetes, and Metabolism

Overview

Endocrinology is the diagnosis and care of disorders of the endocrine system. The principal endocrine problems handled by the general internist include goiter, thyroid nodules, thyroid dysfunction, diabetes mellitus, hyper- and hypocalcemia, adrenal cortex hyper- and hypofunction, endocrine hypertension, gonadal disorders, hyper- and hyponatremia, certain manifestations of pituitary tumors, disorders of mineral metabolism, and hyperlipidemias. Obesity is not strictly an endocrine disorder but is considered part of the spectrum of endocrinology because it frequently enters into the differential diagnosis of endocrine disease and is a major element in the management of non–insulin-dependent diabetes. Prevention efforts focus on complications of hyperlipidemias, obesity, thyroid dysfunction, and diabetes mellitus and on endocrinologic side effects of pharmacologic glucocorticoids and other medications.

The general internist must be able to evaluate and manage common endocrine disorders and refer appropriately. He or she must also be able to evaluate and identify the endocrinologic implications of abnormal serum electrolytes, hypertension, fatigue, and other nonspecific presentations. The general internist plays a key role in managing endocrine emergencies, particularly those encountered in the intensive care unit, including diabetic ketoacidosis and hyperosmolar nonketotic stupor, severe hyper- and hypocalcemia, and addisonian crisis.

Common Clinical Presentations

- Asthenia
- Blood lipid disorders
- Breast discharge
- Change in menstrual, gonadal/sexual function
- Diarrhea
- Disorders of pigmentation
- Goiter (diffuse, nodular)
- Hirsutism
- Hypertension refractory to primary therapy
- Hypotension
- Incidentally discovered abnormalities in serum electrolytes, calcium, phosphate, or glucose
- Mental status changes
- Osteopenia
- Polyuria, polydypsia
- Signs and symptoms of osteopenia
- Symptoms of hyper- and hypoglycemia
- Symptoms of hypermetabolism
- Symptoms of hypometabolism
- Urinary tract stone
- Weight gain, obesity

Procedure Skills
- Dexamethasone suppression test (overnight)
- Home blood glucose monitoring
- ACTH stimulation test

Primary Interpretation of Tests
None specific to the discipline

Ordering and Understanding Tests
- Bone mineral analysis (densitometry)
- Fasting and standardized postprandial serum glucose concentrations
- Glycohemoglobin or serum fructosamine concentration
- Imaging studies of the sella turcica
- Microalbuminuria
- Serum alkaline phosphatase activity (for Paget's disease of bone)
- Serum and urine ketone concentrations (quantitative or qualitative)
- Serum and urine osmolalities
- Serum gonadotropin concentrations (follicle-stimulating hormone, luteinizing hormone)
- Serum lipid profile
- Serum phosphate concentration
- Serum prolactin concentration
- Serum testosterone concentration
- Serum thyroid function tests
- Thyroid scanning and ultrasound
- Urinary calcium, phosphate, uric acid excretion
- Urinary sodium, potassium excretion
- Urine metanephrine, VMA (vanillylmandelic acid), and total catecholamine levels

In-depth knowledge of clinical conditions, including principles of management and indications for referral.

ENDOCRINOLOGY, DIABETES, AND METABOLISM

Competency	Priority		Preferred Learning Venues					
			Outpatient			Inpatient	Didactic	
	FCIM Task Force	Residency Program	Continuity Clinic	Subspecialty Clinic	Other	Other		
Adrenal disorders								
Hypercortisolism	1							
Hypoadrenocortisolism, acute	2							
Hypoadrenocortisolism, chronic	2							
Bone disorders								
Osteopenia/osteoporosis	1							
Paget's disease of bone	2							
Diabetes mellitus								
Diabetic ketoacidosis	1							
Insulin-dependent diabetes	1							
Non–insulin-dependent diabetes	1							
Metabolic disorders								
Hyperosmolar state	1							
Hypoglycemia	1							
Hyponatremia/hypernatremia	1							
Lipid disorders	1							
Obesity	1							
Panhypopituitarism	3							

ENDOCRINOLOGY, DIABETES, AND METABOLISM (CONT.)

Competency	Priority		Preferred Learning Venues					
			Outpatient			Inpatient	Didactic	
	FCIM Task Force	Residency Program	Continuity Clinic	Subspecialty Clinic	Other	Other		
Parathyroid disorders								
Hypercalcemia	1							
Hyperparathyroidism	1							
Hypocalcemia	2							
Reproductive/sexual disorders								
Change in sexual function	1							
Hypogonadism, female menopause	1							
Menstrual disorders	1							
Galactorrhea	2							
Hirsutism/virilization	2							
Hypogonadism, male gonadal failure	2							
Thyroid disorders								
Enlarged thyroid (goiter, nodule)	1							
Hyperthyroidism	1							
Hypothyroidism	1							

Key: 1 = direct patient responsibility preferred; 2 = any form of learning that is centered on a patient; 3 = lectures/seminars/reading suffice.

Gastroenterology and Hepatology

Overview

Gastroenterology encompasses the evaluation and treatment of patients with disorders of the gastrointestinal tract, pancreas, biliary tract, and liver. It includes disorders of organs within the abdominal cavity and requires knowledge of the manifestations of gastrointestinal disorders in other organ systems, such as the skin. Additional areas include knowledge of nutrition and nutritional deficiencies, and screening and prevention, particularly for colorectal cancer.

The general internist should have a wide range of competency in gastroenterology and should be able to provide primary and in some cases secondary preventive care, evaluate a broad array of gastrointestinal symptoms, and manage many gastrointestinal disorders. The general internist is not expected to perform most technical procedures with the important exception of flexible sigmoidoscopy. However, he or she must be familiar with the indications, contraindications, interpretation, and complications of these procedures.

Common Clinical Presentations

- Abdominal distention
- Abdominal pain
- Abnormal liver function tests
- Anorectal discomfort, bleeding, or pruritus
- Anorexia, weight loss
- Ascites
- Constipation
- Diarrhea
- Excess intestinal gas
- Fecal incontinence
- Food intolerance
- Gastrointestinal bleeding
- Heartburn
- Hematemesis
- Indigestion
- Iron-deficiency anemia
- Jaundice
- Liver failure
- Malnutrition
- Melena
- Nausea, vomiting
- Noncardiac chest pain
- Swallowing dysfunction

Procedure Skills
- Flexible sigmoidoscopy
- Paracentesis
- Placement of nasogastric tube
- Sengstaken-Blakemore tube (optional)

Primary Interpretation of Tests
- Fecal leukocytes
- Fecal occult blood test

Ordering and Understanding Tests
- 24-hour esophageal pH monitoring
- Assays for *Helicobacter pylori*
- Bernstein test
- Biopsy of the gastrointestinal mucosa
- Blood tests for autoimmune, cholestatic, genetic liver diseases
- Colonoscopy
- Computed tomography, magnetic resonance imaging, ultrasound of the abdomen
- Contrast studies (including upper gastrointestinal series, small-bowel follow-through, barium enema)
- Stool for ova, parasites
- D-xylose absorption test and other small bowel absorption tests
- Endoscopic retrograde cholangiopancreatography
- Esophageal manometry
- Examination of stool for ova, parasites
- Fecal electrolytes
- Fecal osmolality
- Gall bladder radionuclide scan
- Gastric acid analysis, serum gastrin level, secretin stimulation test
- Viral hepatitis serology
- Lactose and hydrogen breath tests
- Laparoscopy
- Laxative screen
- Liver biopsy
- Mesenteric arteriography
- Percutaneous transhepatic cholangiography
- Qualitative and quantitative, stool fat
- Scans of gastric emptying
- Serum B_{12} and Schilling tests
- Upper endoscopy

In-depth knowledge of clinical conditions, including principles of management and indications for referral.

GASTROENTEROLOGY

Competency	Priority		Preferred Learning Venues					
			Outpatient				Inpatient	Didactic
	FCIM Task Force	Residency Program	Continuity Clinic	Subspecialty Clinic	Other	Other		
Acute abdomen	1							
Acute appendicitis	2							
Ascites	1							
Diarrhea								
Acute	1							
Chronic	1							
Gastroesophageal reflux disease (GERD)								
Uncomplicated GERD	1							
Esophageal stricture	2							
Barrett's esophagus	3							
Gastrointestinal bleeding								
Lower	1							
Occult	1							
Upper	1							
Inflammatory bowel disease	2							
Intestinal disorders								
Diverticulitis	1							
Hemorrhoids	1							
Irritable bowel syndrome	1							
Diverticular abscess	2							
Malabsorption, maldigestion	2							
Mesenteric vascular disease	2							

GASTROENTEROLOGY (CONT.)

Competency	Priority		Preferred Learning Venues				
			Outpatient			Inpatient	Didactic
	FCIM Task Force	Residency Program	Continuity Clinic	Subspecialty Clinic	Other	Other	
Malnutrition	2						
Motility disorders							
Esophagus	1						
Colon	2						
Gastroparesis	2						
Small intestine	3						
Neoplasms							
Cancer (including hepato-biliary)	1						
Colonic polyps	1						
Peptic ulcer disease							
Bleeding ulcer	1						
Helicobacter pylori–induced gastritis	1						
Uncomplicated ulcer	1						
Perforation, obstruction	2						
Peritoneal disease	2						

Key: 1 = direct patient responsibility preferred; 2 = any form of learning that is centered on a patient; 3 = lectures/seminars/reading suffice.

HEPATOLOGY

| Competency | Priority | | Preferred Learning Venues | | | | | |
| | FCIM Task Force | Residency Program | Outpatient | | | Inpatient | Didactic | |
			Continuity Clinic	Subspecialty Clinic	Other	Other		
Biliary tract disease								
Acute cholecystitis	1							
Biliary obstruction	1							
Cholelithiasis	1							
Cholangitis	2							
Cholestatic liver disease								
Primary biliary cirrhosis	3							
Primary sclerosing cholangitis	3							
Cirrhosis (including complications)	1							
Hepatitis								
Drug-induced	1							
Viral	1							
Infiltrative liver diseases								
Other acquired	2							
Inherited	3							
Metabolic	3							
Pancreatitis								
Acute	1							
Chronic	1							

Key: 1 = direct patient responsibility preferred; 2 = any form of learning that is centered on a patient; 3 = lectures/seminars/reading suffice.

Hematology

Overview

The discipline of hematology relates to the care of patients with disorders of the blood, bone marrow, and lymphatic systems, including anemias, hematologic malignancies, and other clonal processes, and congenital and acquired disorders of hemostasis, coagulation, and thrombosis.

The general internist should be competent in 1) the detection of abnormal physical, laboratory, and radiologic findings relating to the lymphohematopoietic system; 2) the assessment of the need for bone marrow aspirate and biopsy and lymph node biopsy; 3) the initial diagnostic evaluation and management of the hemostatic and clotting system; 4) the assessment of the indications and procedure for transfusion of blood and its separate components; 5) the management of therapeutic and prophylactic anticoagulation; 6) the diagnosis and management of common anemias; 7) the pharmacology and use of common chemotherapies; and 8) the management of neutropenia/immunosuppression.

The range of competencies expected for a general internist will vary depending on the availability of a hematologist in the primary care setting. For example, in some communities a general internist may be responsible for bone marrow examination and administration of chemotherapy for certain disorders in conjunction with consultative assistance from appropriate hematologist and pathologist colleagues.

(N.B. Leukemias and lymphomas are found in the Oncology section.)

Common Clinical Presentations

- Abnormalities of peripheral blood smear
- Bleeding, bruising, or petechiae
- Family history of anemia or bleeding disorder
- Lymphadenopathy
- Pallor or fatigue
- Recurrent infections or fever/neutropenia
- Splenomegaly
- Venous or arterial thrombosis, including recurrent thrombosis

Procedure Skills

- Therapeutic phlebotomy
- Bone marrow aspiration and core biopsy (optional)

Primary Interpretation of Tests

- Peripheral blood smear
- Bone marrow aspiration and core biopsy (optional)

Ordering and Understanding Tests

- Bone marrow aspirate, biopsy, and special stains
- Chromosome analysis—peripheral blood and bone marrow
- Clotting assay, including factor levels and mixing studies
- Hemoglobin electrophoresis
- Iron studies
- Lymph node biopsy and lymphoid cell immunophenotype
- Radiologic, sonographic, and nuclear studies to assess adenopathy, splenomegaly, and red cell mass
- Serum and urine electrophoresis
- Vitamin B_{12} levels and Schilling test

In-depth knowledge of clinical conditions, including principles of management and indications for referral.

HEMATOLOGY

Competency	Priority		Preferred Learning Venues				
			Outpatient				
	FCIM Task Force	Residency Program	Continuity Clinic	Subspecialty Clinic	Other	Other	Inpatient	Didactic
Hemochromatosis	2							
Hemostasis and thrombosis								
Abnormal coagulation (abnormal prothrombin and partial thromboplastin times)	1							
Anticardiolipin antibody syndrome	1							
Anticoagulation, fibrinolysis (therapeutic)	1							
Disseminated intravascular coagulation	1							
Hypercoagulable state	2							
Hyperviscosity syndrome	3							
Leukocyte disorders								
Immunosuppression	1							
Neutropenia	1							
Leukemoid reaction	2							
Myeloproliferative disorders								
Chronic myelogenous leukemia	2							
Polycythemia vera	2							

Key: 1 = direct patient responsibility preferred; 2 = any other form of learning that is centered on a patient; 3 = lectures/seminars/reading suffice.

HEMATOLOGY

Competency	Priority		Preferred Learning Venues					
			Outpatient			Inpatient	Didactic	
	FCIM Task Force	Residency Program	Continuity Clinic	Subspecialty Clinic	Other	Other		
Platelet disorders								
Thrombocytopenia	1							
Platelet dysfunction	2							
Thrombocytosis	2							
Polycythemia, secondary	2							
Red cell disorders								
Anemia	1							
Hemoglobinopathy (e.g., sickle cell disease)	1							
Transfusion therapy	1							

Key: 1 = direct patient responsibility preferred; 2 = any other form of learning that is centered on a patient; 3 = lectures/seminars/reading suffice.

Infectious Disease

Overview

Infectious disease medicine requires an understanding of the microbiology, prevention, and management of disorders caused by viral, bacterial, fungal, and parasitic infections, including the appropriate use of antimicrobial agents, vaccines, and other immunobiologic agents. Important elements include the environmental, occupational, and host factors that predispose to infection, as well as basic principles of the epidemiology and transmission of infection.

The general internist should be able to provide appropriate preventive (including optimal use of immunization and chemoprophylaxis), diagnostic, and therapeutic care for most infections. He or she should also be able to evaluate symptoms that may be caused by a wide range of infectious disorders.

General internists should also learn about the diagnostic and management approaches to patients with HIV infection. Experience should include patients with early HIV infection who have few or no symptoms and also patients with advanced HIV infection who manifest the acquired immunodeficiency syndrome (AIDS).

Common Clinical Presentations

- Abdominal or pelvic pain
- Cellulitis
- Cervicitis, vaginal discharge
- Delirium
- Diarrhea
- Dysuria
- Facial or ear pain
- Fever, including fever in immunosuppressed patient
- Hepatitis
- Joint effusion
- Limb, sacral ulcers
- Lymphadenopathy
- Meningitis
- Penile discharge
- Prevention, public health concerns (immunization, susceptibility and exposure, prophylaxis)
- Productive cough, pulmonary infiltrate
- Rash (cellulitis, erythema, petechiae, purpura, tinea)
- Red eye
- Skin abscess
- Sore throat, painful swallowing
- Vomiting

Counseling Skills
- Alternative health practices
- HIV risk assessment
- Post-diagnosis counseling
- Substance abuse

Procedure Skills
- Incision and drainage of superficial abscesses
- Proper collection of culture specimens from throat, cervix, vagina, rectum, urethra, and blood
- Saline and potassium hydroxide preparation of vaginal fluid, skin scrapings
- Tuberculin and anergy panel skin tests

Primary Interpretation of Tests
None specific to the discipline

Ordering and Understanding Tests
- Antibiotic sensitivity testing and serum levels
- Biopsy of tissues
- CD4 lymphocyte counts
- Cerebrospinal fluid cell count, chemistry, VDRL, cryptococcal antigen, cytology
- Computed tomography, magnetic resonance imaging of the central nervous system
- ELISA, polymerase chain reaction, and immunoblotting techniques
- Induced sputum stain for *Pneumocystis carinii*
- Polymerase chain reaction, ELISA, and Western blot for detection of infectious diseases
- Serology for infections (e.g., Lyme disease, syphilis, etc.)
- Syphilis serology and dark-field microscopy
- Toxoplasma serology

In-depth knowledge of clinical conditions, including principles of management and indications for referral.

INFECTIOUS DISEASE

| Competency | Priority | | Preferred Learning Venues | | | | | |
| | FCIM Task Force | Residency Program | Outpatient | | | Inpatient | Didactic |
			Continuity Clinic	Subspecialty Clinic	Other		
Central nervous system							
Meningitis	1						
Encephalitis	2						
Conjunctivitis	1						
Endocarditis	1						
Fever of unknown origin	1						
Fungal (histoplasmosis, coccidioidomycosis)	3						
Gastrointestinal							
Biliary tract infection	1						
Gastroenteritis	1						
Infectious diarrhea	1						
Viral hepatitis	1						
Peritonitis	2						
Genitourinary							
Cervicitis, vaginitis	1						
Common sexually transmitted diseases (gonorrhea, chlamydia, trichomonas, herpes simplex, syphilis)	1						
Pelvic inflammatory disease	1						
Prostatitis, epididymitis	1						
Urethritis	1						
Urinary tract infection	1						

Key: 1 = direct patient responsibility preferred; 2 = any other form of learning that is centered on a patient; 3 = lectures/seminars/reading suffice.

INFECTIOUS DISEASE (CONT.)

Competency	Priority		Preferred Learning Venues					
			Outpatient			Inpatient	Didactic	
	FCIM Task Force	Residency Program	Continuity Clinic	Subspecialty Clinic	Other	Other		
HIV disease (*see* HIV Infection)								
Infection in the immuno-suppressed patient	1							
Lyme disease	2							
Malaria	3							
Otitis	1							
Respiratory								
Acute epiglottitis, pharyngitis	1							
Pneumonia (community and nosocomial), bronchitis	1							
Sinusitis	1							
Upper respiratory infection	1							
Empyema	2							
Rheumatologic/musculoskeletal								
Osteomyelitis	2							
Septic arthritis	2							
Sepsis, septic shock syndrome	1							
Skin infections								
Cellulitis	1							
Ulcers	1							

INFECTIOUS DISEASE (CONT.)

Competency	Priority		Preferred Learning Venues					
			Outpatient			Inpatient	Didactic	
	FCIM Task Force	Residency Program	Continuity Clinic	Subspecialty Clinic	Other	Other		
Tuberculosis								
Active infection	1							
Positive tuberculin skin test	1							
Viral								
Herpes simplex infection	1							
Influenza	1							
Mononucleosis	1							
Varicella zoster infection	2							
Cytomegalovirus	3							

Key: 1 = direct patient responsibility preferred; 2 = any other form of learning that is centered on a patient; 3 = lectures/seminars/reading suffice.

HIV INFECTION

Competency	Priority		Preferred Learning Venues					
			Outpatient			Inpatient	Other	Didactic
	FCIM Task Force	Residency Program	Continuity Clinic	Subspecialty Clinic	Other			
General management								
Evaluation and management of early disease								
Advance directives evaluation	1							
Assessment of social support systems	1							
Monitoring progression to AIDS	1							
Assessment of alternative health practices	2							
Ongoing staging								
Diagnosing AIDS-defining opportunistic infections	1							
Functional assessment	1							
Mental status evaluation	1							
Nutritional assessment	1							
Referral to case-management agencies	1							
Palliative and terminal care	1							
Pregnancy counseling (pretest, post-test, risk factors)	3							
Gynecologic complications								
Vaginal candidiasis	1							
Cervical dysplasia/neoplasia	2							
Pelvic inflammatory disease	2							

HIV INFECTION (CONT.)

Competency	Priority		Preferred Learning Venues					
	FCIM Task Force	Residency Program	Outpatient			Other	Inpatient	Didactic
			Continuity Clinic	Subspecialty Clinic	Other			
Infectious diseases (see also *Preventive measures* below and specific organ-based complications)								
Mycobacterial disease	1							
Pneumocystis carinii pneumonia	1							
Cytomegalovirus disease	2							
Syphilis (diagnosis, treatment)	2							
Oral complications	1							
Preventive measures								
Antibiotic prophylaxis								
Pneumocystis carinii pneumonia	1							
Tuberculosis	1							
Antiretroviral drug therapy	1							
Immunizations	1							
Transmission of HIV	1							
Mycobacterium avium complex	2							
Protease inhibitor therapy	2							
Toxoplasmosis	2							
AIDS-defining malignancies								
Kaposi's sarcoma	2							
Non-Hodgkin's lymphoma	2							
Squamous cell carcinoma (cervix or anus)	3							

Key: 1 = direct patient responsibility preferred; 2 = any other form of learning that is centered on a patient; 3 = lectures/seminars/reading suffice.

HIV INFECTION (CONT.)

Competency	Priority		Preferred Learning Venues					
	FCIM Task Force	Residency Program	Outpatient			Inpatient	Didactic	
			Continuity Clinic	Subspecialty Clinic	Other	Other		
Dermatologic complications								
Kaposi's sarcoma	2							
Scabies, folliculitis	2							
Seborrheic dermatitis	2							
Bacillary angiomatosis	3							
Gastrointestinal complications								
Diarrhea	1							
Esophageal candidiasis	2							
Esophageal ulcer disease	2							
Hepatomegaly, hepatitis, jaundice	2							
Wasting syndrome	2							
Neurologic complications								
Dementia	1							
Central nervous system mass lesions	2							
Cryptococcal meningitis	2							
Neurosyphilis	2							

Key: 1 = direct patient responsibility preferred; 2 = any other form of learning that is centered on a patient; 3 = lectures/seminars/reading suffice.

Nephrology

Overview

Nephrology involves disease of the kidneys, its contiguous collecting system, and its vasculature. The kidneys play a key role in fluid, electrolyte, and acid-base regulation and are affected by a wide range of systemic disorders, drugs, and toxins.

The general internist should be competent to evaluate and appropriately refer patients with glomerular disorders, asymptomatic urine abnormalities, tubulo-interstitial diseases, renal vascular disease, renal failure, nephrolithiasis, tubular defects, and infections and neoplasms of the kidneys, bladder, and urethra, and should also be able to provide principal treatment for some of these conditions. He or she should be able to manage fluid, electrolyte, and acid-base disorders; understand the ways in which systemic diseases may affect the kidneys; and recognize the potential nephrotoxicity of various therapeutic and diagnostic agents. The general internist must also be familiar with guidelines for pre-dialysis management of patients with renal failure and be able to recognize indications for dialysis and for referral to a nephrologist.

The range of competencies in managing renal disease will depend on the availability of a nephrologist to the primary care internist. Although all general internists should know the indications for dialysis, in some cases (for example, if a nephrologist is unavailable), the general internist may be responsible for initiating and maintaining patients on peritoneal dialysis. In most situations, hemodialysis will be the responsibility of a nephrologist, as will renal biopsies and nephrostomy tube placement.

Common Clinical Presentations

- Abnormalities noted on urinalysis (including proteinuria, hematuria, bacteriuria, pyuria, and cylinduria)
- Complaints referable to bladder outlet (urgency, hesitancy)
- Dysuria
- Edema
- Flank or suprapubic pain or tenderness
- Frequency and complaints referable to increased or decreased urine volume
- Hematuria (gross)
- Hypertension
- Incontinence
- Presenting features of uremia
- Renal colic
- Renal mass or bruit

Procedure Skills
- Calculation of creatinine clearance
- Calculation of fractional excretion of sodium
- Peritoneal cavity aspiration per indwelling dialysis catheter
- Femoral temporary hemodialysis catheter placement (optional)
- Peritoneal dialysis catheterization (optional)
- Suprapubic bladder catheterization (optional)

Primary Interpretation of Tests
None specific to the discipline

Ordering and Understanding Tests
- 24-hour urine excretion of calcium, oxalate, citrate, uric acid, and protein
- Computed tomography, magnetic resonance imaging, and angiography, and ultrasound of the kidneys
- Creatinine clearance
- Cystometrography
- Cystoscopy
- Fractional excretion of sodium
- Intravenous pyelography
- Radionuclide renal scan
- Renal angiography and venography
- Renal biopsy
- Retrograde pyelography
- Serologic tests for evaluating glomerulonephritis
- Urinary calculus analysis
- Urine electrolytes (sodium, potassium, chloride)
- Urine/plasma osmolality

In-depth knowledge of clinical conditions, including principles of management and indications for referral.

NEPHROLOGY

Competency	Priority		Preferred Learning Venues					
			Outpatient			Other	Inpatient	Didactic
	FCIM Task Force	Residency Program	Continuity Clinic	Subspecialty Clinic	Other			
Acid-base disorders	1							
Acute renal failure								
Acute (ischemic) tubular necrosis	1							
Drug-induced (radiocontrast, analgesics, etc.)	1							
Interstitial	2							
Atheroembolic	3							
Chronic renal failure								
Conservative management (before dialysis)	1							
Hemodialysis	2							
Peritoneal dialysis	2							
Transplantation	3							
Fluid and electrolyte disorders	1							
Glomerular diseases								
Acute glomerulonephritis	1							
Chronic glomerulonephritis	1							
Nephrotic syndrome	1							
Hypertension								
Hypertensive crisis	1							
Secondary hypertension	1							

Key: 1 = direct patient responsibility preferred; 2 = any form of learning that is centered on a patient; 3 = lectures/seminars/reading suffice.

NEPHROLOGY (CONT.)

Competency	Priority		Preferred Learning Venues					
			Outpatient					
	FCIM Task Force	Residency Program	Continuity Clinic	Subspecialty Clinic	Other	Other	Inpatient	Didactic
Inherited diseases								
Polycystic kidneys	3							
Kidney disease in systemic illness								
Diabetes mellitus	1							
Hypertension	1							
Other systemic diseases	2							
Neoplasia								
Bladder carcinoma	2							
Renal cell carcinoma	2							
Nephrolithiasis								
Diagnosis of renal stone disease	1							
Management of acute renal colic	1							
Obstructive uropathy	1							
Urinary tract infection								
Cystitis	1							
Pyelonephritis	1							

NEPHROLOGY (CONT.)

Competency	Priority		Preferred Learning Venues					
	FCIM Task Force	Residency Program	Outpatient			Inpatient	Didactic
			Continuity Clinic	Subspecialty Clinic	Other	Other		
Urologic disorders								
Cancer of the prostate (detection)	1							
Erectile dysfunction	1							
Incontinence	1							
Prostate disease	1							
Bladder outlet obstruction	2							

Key: 1 = direct patient responsibility preferred; 2 = any form of learning that is centered on a patient; 3 = lectures/seminars/reading suffice.

Neurology

Overview

Neurology encompasses the prevention and management of disorders of the central and peripheral nervous systems. Other conditions, such as headache, may be caused by non-neural dysfunction but are often considered under the category of neurology.

The general internist should possess a broad range of competency in neurology. He or she should be able to perform and interpret a detailed neurologic examination; should be competent in the primary and secondary prevention of neurologic diseases; and should be familiar with the presenting features, diagnosis, and treatment of common neurologic disorders.

The general internist may encounter neurologic disorders in various settings, including ambulatory care, hospital, long-term care, and home care. In communities where a neurologist is not available, the general internist may be a consultant for some complex neurologic disorders (for example, control of status epilepticus).

Common Clinical Presentations

- Abnormal speech
- Abnormal vision
- Altered sensation
- Confusion
- Disturbed gait or coordination
- Dizziness, vertigo
- Headache
- Hearing loss
- Localized pain syndromes: facial pain, radiculopathy
- Loss of consciousness
- Memory impairment
- Seizure
- Sleep disorder
- Tremor
- Weakness/paresis (generalized, localized)

Procedure Skills

- Caloric stimulation test
- Tensilon (edrophonium chloride) test (optional)

Ordering and Understanding Tests
- Anticonvulsant drug levels
- Carotid Doppler echo scans
- Computed tomography, magnetic resonance imaging of central nervous system
- Digital intravenous angiography
- Electroencephalography, evoked potentials (visual, auditory, sensory)
- Electromyography, nerve conduction studies
- Muscle biopsy
- Myelography
- Screen for toxins, heavy metals
- Sleep study

In-depth knowledge of clinical conditions, including principles of management and indications for referral.

NEUROLOGY

| Competency | Priority | | Preferred Learning Venues | | | | |
| | FCIM Task Force | Residency Program | Outpatient | | | Inpatient | Didactic |
			Continuity Clinic	Subspecialty Clinic	Other	Other	
Benign positional vertigo	1						
Central nervous system infection							
Meningitis	1						
Encephalitis	2						
Brain abscess	3						
Cerebrovascular disease							
Stroke	1						
Transient ischemic attack	1						
Dementias	1						
Epidural abscess	2						
Epilepsy	1						
Headache (especially migraine)	1						
Labyrynthitis	2						
Lumbar, cervical disk syndromes	1						

NEUROLOGY (CONT.)

| Competency | Priority | | Preferred Learning Venues | | | | | |
| | FCIM Task Force | Residency Program | Outpatient | | | Inpatient | | Didactic |
			Continuity Clinic	Subspecialty Clinic	Other	Other		
Multiple sclerosis	2							
Neuromuscular disease								
Myopathy	2							
Amyotrophy	3							
Guillain-Barré syndrome	3							
Muscular dystrophy	3							
Myasthenia gravis	3							
Parkinson's disease	2							
Peripheral neuropathy	2							
Sleep disorders	1							
Subarachnoid hemorrhage	2							
Subdural hematoma	2							
Toxic encephalopathies (e.g., alcohol withdrawal)	1							

Key: 1 = direct patient responsibility preferred; 2 = any form of learning that is centered on a patient; 3 = lectures/seminars/reading suffice.

Oncology

Overview

Medical oncology is the diagnosis and management of benign and malignant neoplasms. The general internist should have a wide range of competencies in the evaluation and management of neoplastic disease. He or she must be able to 1) identify patients at risk for malignancy and counsel them regarding risk reduction and screening; 2) investigate clinical syndromes suggestive of underlying malignancy; 3) undertake the palliative care of patients with common solid and hematologic tumors; 4) identify neoplasms with a potential for cure and direct affected patients to the appropriate centers or providers; and 5) participate in the difficult decisions regarding all aspects of management, including diagnostic evaluation and screening, treatment, and palliative care. In addition, the general internist must be familiar with the administration, side effects, and drug interactions of therapeutic agents commonly used for the treatment of malignant disease.

Whether a generalist assumes full responsibility for any or all of these functions will depend on the clinical setting of his or her practice. The general internist should seek subspecialty consultation early in the care of patients with malignant disease who may be candidates for aggressive treatment with curative intent.

Common Clinical Presentations

- Anemia
- Ascites
- Bleeding
- Bowel obstruction
- Cough, hoarseness, hemoptysis
- Lymphadenopathy, soft tissue mass
- Organ enlargement, mass
- Pleural or peritoneal effusion of unknown cause
- Sensory polyneuropathy
- Superior vena cava syndrome
- Weight loss

Procedure Skills

- Bone marrow aspiration and biopsy (optional)
- Fine-needle aspiration of thyroid and breast (optional)
- Intrathecal chemotherapy (optional)

Primary Interpretation of Tests

None specific to the discipline

Ordering and Understanding Tests
- Biopsy
- Bone marrow cytogenetics, immunophenotyping
- Cytology and pathology
- Diagnostic and interventional radiology
- DNA content and molecular markers of tumor tissue
- Estrogen and progesterone receptors
- Fiberoptic examinations
- Imaging studies, including computed tomography and magnetic resonance imaging nuclear studies
- Serologic markers for tumors
- Ultrasound

In-depth knowledge of clinical conditions, including principles of management and indications for referral.

ONCOLOGY

| Competency | Priority | | Preferred Learning Venues | | | | |
| | FCIM Task Force | Residency Program | Outpatient | | | Inpatient | Didactic |
			Continuity Clinic	Subspecialty Clinic	Other		
Advance planning and management of end-of-life issues	1						
Breast cancer (pre- and post-menopausal)	1						
Dermatologic							
Basal cell carcinoma	1						
Melanoma	1						
Actinic keratosis	2						
Squamous cell carcinoma	2						
Gastrointestinal							
Cancer of the colon, rectum	1						
Cancer of the anus	2						
Cancer of the esophagus	2						
Cancer of the pancreas	2						
Cancer of the stomach	2						
Hepatoma	2						
Metastatic disease to various sites	2						
Cancer of the gallbladder, bile ducts	3						

ONCOLOGY (CONT.)

| Competency | Priority | | Preferred Learning Venues | | | | | |
	FCIM Task Force	Residency Program	Continuity Clinic	Subspecialty Clinic	Other	Other	Inpatient	Didactic
				Outpatient				
Genitourinary								
Cervical dysplasia and cancer	1							
Prostate cancer	1							
Endometrial cancer	2							
Kidney cancer	2							
Ovarian cancer	2							
Testicular cancer	2							
Ureter, bladder cancer	2							
Head and neck								
Cancer of the head, neck	2							
Cancer of the thyroid	2							
Cancer of the parathyroid	3							
Hematologic malignancies and lymphoma								
Chronic lymphocytic leukemia	1							
Hodgkin's and non-Hodgkin's lymphomas	1							
Leukemia, acute	2							
Multiple myeloma	2							
Myelodysplastic syndrome	2							
Management of pain, emesis, and nutrition	1							

Key: 1 = direct patient responsibility preferred; 2 = any form of learning that is centered on a patient; 3 = lectures/seminars/reading suffice.

ONCOLOGY (CONT.)

Competency	Priority		Preferred Learning Venues					
			Outpatient			Other	Inpatient	Didactic
	FCIM Task Force	Residency Program	Continuity Clinic	Subspecialty Clinic	Other			
Neurologic								
CNS lymphoma	2							
Metastatic disease to the CNS	2							
Primary brain tumors	2							
Oncologic emergencies								
Depressed CNS function due to brain malignancy	1							
Hypercalcemia	1							
Pericardial tamponade	1							
Renal failure due to ureteral obstruction	2							
Spinal cord compression	2							
Tumor lysis syndrome	2							
Pulmonary								
Cancer of the lung	1							
Superior vena cava syndrome	1							
Mediastinal tumors	2							
Pleural malignancy	2							
Bronchial carcinoid	3							

Key: 1 = direct patient responsibility preferred; 2 = any form of learning that is centered on a patient; 3 = lectures/seminars/reading suffice.

Ophthalmology

Overview

Ophthalmology is the branch of medicine that investigates and treats disorders of the eye. The ophthalmologist is concerned with visual function and with infectious, inflammatory, traumatic, degenerative, and neoplastic disorders.

The general internist must be able to evaluate many ophthalmologic complaints, including pain, redness, itching, and visual changes. He or she should be able to identify and treat frequently encountered problems, such as conjunctivitis, and identify problems requiring referral. These functions require competency in the office examination of vision and the eye, an appreciation of the critical elements in a patient's history, and an understanding of the indications for routine and emergency referral.

In addition, the general internist must be able to recognize the funduscopic findings of systemic illness, including hypertension and diabetes mellitus, and realize that ocular complaints may herald other illness.

Common Clinical Presentations

- Acute or chronic loss of vision
- Cataracts
- Common disorders of the eyelid
- Elevated intraocular pressure
- Exophthalmos
- Floaters and visual phenomena
- Funduscopic abnormalities (papilledema, hemorrhage, exudate)
- Injuries
- Pain
- Red eye

Procedure Skills

- Fluorescein stain of the cornea
- Bandaging and patching (optional)
- Eye irrigation (optional)
- Removal of superficial foreign body (optional)
- Slit lamp examination (optional)

Ordering and Understanding Tests

- Fluorescein angiography
- Formal visual field testing
- Intraocular pressure testing
- Slit lamp examination

In-depth knowledge of clinical conditions, including principles of management and indications for referral.

OPHTHALMOLOGY

Competency	Priority		Preferred Learning Venues					
			Outpatient			Inpatient	Other	Didactic
	FCIM Task Force	Residency Program	Continuity Clinic	Subspecialty Clinic	Other			
Blepharitis	1							
Cataracts	1							
Chlamydial infection	3							
Conjunctivitis	1							
Corneal abrasions	1							
Corneal infection	3							
Detachment of retina or vitreous	2							
Dry eye syndromes	1							
Foreign bodies, external and superficial	2							
Glaucoma	1							
Herpes zoster ophthalmicus	2							
Hordeolum, chalazion	1							
Keratitis, corneal ulcer	3							
Macular degeneration	1							
Optic atrophy	3							
Optic neuritis	2							
Orbital or periorbital cellulitis	2							

OPHTHALMOLOGY (CONT.)

Competency	Priority		Preferred Learning Venues					
			Outpatient			Inpatient	Other	Didactic
	FCIM Task Force	Residency Program	Continuity Clinic	Subspecialty Clinic	Other			
Pinguecula, pterygium	2							
Retinal artery or vein occlusion	3							
Scleritis, episcleritis	2							
Subconjunctival hemorrhage	1							
Trauma (orbital fracture, hyphema)	3							
Uveitis	2							

Key: 1 = direct patient responsibility preferred; 2 = any form of learning that is centered on a patient; 3 = lectures/seminars/reading suffice.

Otolaryngology

Overview

Otolaryngology involves the diagnosis and management of disorders of the ears, nose, and throat. The general internist should be able to evaluate and manage such common disorders as pharyngitis, otitis, and sinusitis and recognize more complicated conditions that require subspecialty consultation. He or she should play a key role in screening for and prevention of aerodigestive tract malignancies, which occur particularly often in patients who smoke. The general internist should also be competent in evaluating such specific symptoms as hoarseness, hearing loss, and facial pain.

Common Clinical Presentations

Ears

- Discharge
- Hearing loss
- Pain
- Tinnitus
- Vertigo

Nose

- Airway obstruction
- Congestion or discharge, sneezing
- Epistaxis
- Facial or sinus pain
- Nocturnal airway obstruction, sleep apnea
- Snoring

Throat

- Cervical adenopathy
- Hoarseness
- Oral lesions
- Sore throat

Procedure Skills

Ears

- Insertion of wick in auditory canal
- Removal of cerumen

Nose

- Anterior nasal packing
- Speculum rhinoscopy
- Transillumination of maxillary sinuses

Throat

- Indirect laryngoscopy (optional)

Primary Interpretation of Tests

Nose
- Waters' view radiograph of sinuses

Ordering and Understanding Tests

Ears
- Audiometry

Nose
- Aeroallergen skin sensitivity testing
- Limited computed tomography of the sinuses
- Radiography of the sinuses

Throat
- Culture
- Polysomnography
- Rapid streptococcal antigen test

In-depth knowledge of clinical conditions, including principles of management and indications for referral.

OTOLARYNGOLOGY

Competency	Priority		Preferred Learning Venues					
			Outpatient			Inpatient	Didactic	
	FCIM Task Force	Residency Program	Continuity Clinic	Subspecialty Clinic	Other	Other		
Ears								
Benign positional vertigo	1							
Cerumen impaction	1							
Otitis	1							
Sensorineural hearing loss	1							
Acute labyrinthitis	2							
Eustachian tube dysfunction	2							
Nose								
Epistaxis	1							
Rhinitis, allergic	1							
Sinusitis	1							
Nasal polyps	2							
Rhinitis, vasomotor	2							
Septal deviation	2							
Rhinitis, medicamentosa	3							

OTOLARYNGOLOGY (CONT.)

Competency	Priority		Preferred Learning Venues					
	FCIM Task Force	Residency Program	Outpatient			Inpatient	Didactic
			Continuity Clinic	Subspecialty Clinic	Other		
Throat							
Laryngitis	1						
Masses or lesions of the oral cavity	1						
Pharyngitis	1						
Sleep apnea	1						
Peritonsillar abscess	2						
Acute epiglottitis	3						

Key: 1 = direct patient responsibility preferred; 2 = any form of learning that is centered on a patient; 3 = lectures/seminars/reading suffice.

Psychiatry

Overview

Psychiatry refers to the prevention and treatment of mental disorders and associated emotional, behavioral, and stress-related problems. In general internal medicine practice, management of risk factors for mental disorders and early diagnosis and intervention for established disease (primary and secondary prevention) are important elements. The general internist should have a wide range of competency in psychiatric disease, particularly as it is encountered in outpatient settings and should be able to diagnose symptoms and use pharmacotherapy, behavioral modification, and counseling to provide primary and secondary preventive care and initially manage many mental disorders.

Patients hospitalized for general medical problems and those in the intensive care unit may have significant psychiatric comorbidity that contributes to general medical morbidity and length of stay. In these and all other settings, the general internist must be able to evaluate and manage psychiatric comorbidity effectively with appropriate specialty consultation.

The range of competencies expected of a general internist will depend on the availability of psychiatrists in the primary practice setting. In some communities, the general internist may be responsible for both initial and maintenance psychopharmacologic management of many mental disorders. Refractory cases and patients with mental disorders requiring psychotherapeutic interventions will generally be referred to a mental health professional, as will patients who are suicidal, psychotic, or dangerous and those in need of psychiatric hospitalization.

Common Clinical Presentations
- Agitation or excitement
- Anxiety
- Confusion
- Delusions or bizarre beliefs
- Depressed or sad mood
- Fatigue
- Hallucinations
- Insomnia
- Memory loss
- Poor hygiene or self-care
- Strange speech or behavior
- Suicide risk
- Suspiciousness or feelings of persecution
- Unexplained changes in personality or performance
- Unexplained physical symptoms suggesting somatization

Procedure Skills
- Depression inventory
- Mental status examination, including standardized cognitive examinations (e.g., Mini-Mental State Exam) when indicated

Ordering and Understanding Tests
- Electroencephalography
- Neuropsychologic evaluation

In-depth knowledge of clinical conditions, including principles of management and indications for referral.

PSYCHIATRY

Competency	Priority		Preferred Learning Venues					
			Outpatient			Inpatient	Didactic	
	FCIM Task Force	Residency Program	Continuity Clinic	Subspecialty Clinic	Other			Other
Adjustment disorders (grief, life-cycle changes)	1							
Anxiety disorders	2							
Bipolar disorder	2							
Cognitive disorders	2							
Delirium	1							
Dementia	1							
Dissociative disorders	3							
Eating disorders	1							
Major depression, dysthymia	1							
Panic disorders	1							
Personality disorders	2							
Schizophrenia	2							
Sexual dysfunction	1							
Sleep disorders	1							
Somatization	1							

Key: 1 = direct patient responsibility preferred; 2 = any other form of learning that is centered on a patient; 3 = lectures/seminars/reading suffice.

Pulmonary Medicine

Overview

Pulmonary medicine is the diagnosis and management of disorders of the lungs, upper airways, thoracic cavity, and chest wall. The pulmonary specialist has expertise in neoplastic, inflammatory, and infectious disorders of the lung parenchyma, pleura, and airways; pulmonary vascular disease and its effect on the cardiovascular system; and detection and prevention of occupational and environmental causes of lung disease. Other specialized areas include respiratory failure and sleep-disordered breathing.

The general internist should be able to evaluate and manage cough, dyspnea, fever with infiltrates, mass or nodule on the chest radiograph, pleurisy, and pleural effusion. He or she should also be able to diagnose and manage patients with common respiratory infections; initiate the diagnostic evaluation of respiratory neoplasm; and manage the initial approach to patients with respiratory failure, including those in intensive care units.

The internist will usually be assisted by the pulmonary specialist for diagnostic procedures and complicated conditions such as advanced respiratory failure. If such expertise is not available, the internist, with additional training, may have to assume these roles.

Common Clinical Presentations

- Chest pain
- Cough
- Dyspnea
- Excessive daytime sleepiness
- Febrile patient with infiltrate
- Hemoptysis
- Nodule or mass on chest radiograph
- Pleural effusion, pleurisy
- Stridor, hoarseness
- Wheezing

Procedure Skills (*see also* Critical Care Medicine)

- Arterial blood gas sampling
- Endotracheal intubation
- Monitoring of oxygen saturation
- Skin test for anergy, tuberculosis
- Spirometry and peak flow assessment
- Pulmonary artery catheterization
- Thoracentesis
- Pleural biopsy (optional)

Primary Interpretation of Tests

- Complete pulmonary function tests (spirometry; measurement of lung volumes, diffusing capacity, flow volume loop)
- Pulmonary artery catheter readings

Ordering and Understanding Tests

- Bronchoscopy, including lavage and biopsy
- Cardiopulmonary exercise test
- Computed tomography of thorax
- Cytology, pathology of lung and pleural biopsy specimens
- Diagnostic studies for venous thrombosis
- Mediastinoscopy, mediastinotomy
- Pleural fluid analysis
- Pulmonary angiography
- Sleep study
- Ventilation/perfusion lung scans

In-depth knowledge of clinical conditions, including principles of management and indications for referral.

PULMONARY MEDICINE

Competency	Priority		Preferred Learning Venues					
			Outpatient					
	FCIM Task Force	Residency Program	Continuity Clinic	Subspecialty Clinic	Other	Other	Inpatient	Didactic
Adult respiratory distress syndrome	1							
Airways disease								
Asthma	1							
Bronchitis	1							
Chronic obstructive pulmonary disease	1							
Upper airway obstruction	1							
Bronchiectasis	2							
Aspiration pneumonia	1							
Congenital lung disease								
Cystic fibrosis	2							
Alpha$_1$-antitrypsin deficiency	3							
Dysmotile cilia syndrome	3							

Key: 1 = direct patient responsibility preferred; 2 = any other form of learning that is centered on a patient; 3 = lectures/seminars/reading suffice.

PULMONARY MEDICINE (CONT.)

| Competency | Priority | | Preferred Learning Venues | | | | |
| | FCIM Task Force | Residency Program | Outpatient | | | Inpatient | Didactic |
			Continuity Clinic	Subspecialty Clinic	Other	Other	
Infection							
Pneumonia							
Community-acquired	1						
Hospital-acquired	1						
In immunosuppressed patient	1						
Atypical mycobacteria	2						
Empyema	2						
Lung abscess	2						
Pulmonary mycoses	2						
Tuberculosis	2						
Interstitial disease							
Drug-induced	2						
Hypersensitivity	2						
Idiopathic pulmonary fibrosis	2						
Sarcoidosis	2						
Collagen vascular disease	3						
Eosinophilic pneumonia	3						
Neoplasia							
Confirmed lung cancer	1						
Solitary nodule	1						
Mediastinal	2						

PULMONARY MEDICINE (CONT.)

Competency	Priority		Preferred Learning Venues					
			Outpatient			Inpatient	Didactic	
	FCIM Task Force	Residency Program	Continuity Clinic	Subspecialty Clinic	Other	Other		
Occupational disease								
Asbestos-related	3							
Occupational asthma	3							
Pneumoconiosis	3							
Pleuritis/pleural disease								
Pleural effusion	1							
Pneumothorax	1							
Neoplastic	2							
Non-neoplastic	2							
Prevention								
Avoidance of respiratory irritants, allergens	1							
Immunization	1							
Smoking cessation	1							
Pulmonary carcinogens (radon, passive smoking)	2							
Pulmonary disease in pregnancy	2							
Sleep-disordered breathing	1							
Vascular lung disease								
Pulmonary hypertension								
Cor pulmonale	1							
Primary	3							
Thromboembolism	1							
Vasculitis (Wegener's, pulmonary/renal syndromes)	2							

Key: 1 = direct patient responsibility preferred; 2 = any other form of learning that is centered on a patient; 3 = lectures/seminars/reading suffice.

Rheumatology

Overview

Rheumatology and nonoperative (office) orthopedics deal with the prevention, diagnosis, and management of crystalline diseases, systemic rheumatic diseases, spondyloarthropathies, vasculitis, inflammatory muscle disease, osteoporosis, osteoarthritis, recreational and sports injury, and soft-tissue diseases and trauma. The goal of rheumatology is early diagnosis and treatment of these conditions to prevent disability and death.

The general internist needs to have competency in the initial diagnosis and management of acute arthritis and musculoskeletal disorders and in the long-term care of systemic disorders. He or she must also be proficient in monitoring the effects of anti-inflammatory, immunosuppressive, and cytotoxic drugs.

Common Clinical Presentations

- Joint pain and/or swelling (acute or chronic, monoarticular or polyarticular)
- Muscle aches (localized or diffuse)
- Musculoskeletal weakness
- Nonarticular signs and symptoms of rheumatologic disease, e.g., Raynaud's phenomenon and skin rash
- Regional pain of the neck, shoulder, lower back, hip, knee, hands, or wrists
- Traumatic joint

Procedure Skills

- Therapeutic injection of corticosteroid and arthrocentesis for the knee joint
- Therapeutic injection of corticosteroid to the periarticular structures (bursal) of the shoulder, knee, elbow, and foot
- Arthrocentesis of other joints (optional)

Primary Interpretation of Tests

- Analysis of synovial fluid
- Plain bone radiographs of joints and spine

Ordering and Understanding Tests

- Anti-DNA, anti-Sm, anti-RNP, and anti-SS-A antibodies
- Antineutrophil cytoplasmic antibody (ANCA)
- Complement level
- Erythrocyte sedimentation rate
- Fluorescent antinuclear antibody (ANA)
- Rheumatoid factor
- Synovial analysis for crystals

In-depth knowledge of clinical conditions, including principles of management and indications for referral.

RHEUMATOLOGY

Competency	Priority		Preferred Learning Venues					
			Outpatient					
	FCIM Task Force	Residency Program	Continuity Clinic	Subspecialty Clinic	Other	Other	Inpatient	Didactic
Crystal-induced synovitis	1							
Degenerative joint disease	1							
Fibromyalgia	1							
Inflammatory myopathy	2							
Occupational/sports-related overuse syndromes								
Achilles tendonitis	1							
Iliotibial band	1							
Lateral epicondylitis	1							
Plantar fasciitis	1							
Rotator cuff tendonitis	1							
Trochanteric bursitis	1							
Osteomyelitis	2							
Osteoporosis and complications	1							
Polymyalgia rheumatica	2							

Key: 1 = direct patient responsibility preferred; 2 = any other form of learning that is centered on a patient; 3 = lectures/seminars/reading suffice.

RHEUMATOLOGY (CONT.)

Competency	Priority		Preferred Learning Venues					
			Outpatient			Inpatient	Other	Didactic
	FCIM Task Force	Residency Program	Continuity Clinic	Subspecialty Clinic	Other			
Regional pain syndromes								
Acute or chronic bursitis (hip, shoulder, knee)	1							
Acute or chronic tendonitis (shoulder, elbow, wrist)	1							
Back, neck pain	1							
Foot pain	1							
Rheumatoid arthritis	1							
Scleroderma	2							
Septic arthritis								
Gonococcal	2							
Nongonococcal	2							
Seronegative spondyloarthritis	2							
Systemic lupus erythematosus	1							
Vasculitis								
Temporal (granulomatous)	2							
Polyarteritis and hypersensitivity angiitis	3							

Key: 1 = direct patient responsibility preferred; 2 = any other form of learning that is centered on a patient; 3 = lectures/seminars/reading suffice.

THE CLINICAL COMPETENCIES

Site-Specific Clinical Competencies

- Consultative Medicine

- Critical Care Medicine

- Emergency Medicine

Consultative Medicine

Overview

As much as one third of a general internist's time may be spent in the role of consultant. Although much of this activity has traditionally been centered on care of hospitalized patients undergoing surgery, it also includes outpatient preoperative evaluation and management of medical conditions in pregnant women and in patients with psychiatric disease. As consultant, the internist frequently has a central role in the overall management of the patient's medical care by coordinating subspecialists' recommendations and assuring long-term follow-up.

General internists should have an appreciation of the body of knowledge that has developed in consultative medicine. Most important is an understanding of the physiologic response to surgery and anesthesia, disease-related and procedure-related risk, prophylactic therapy to prevent perioperative problems, and postoperative medical complications. The general internist should also sufficiently understand the physiology of pregnancy and the categories of psychiatric disease and its pharmacologic treatment to manage medical problems in these patients effectively.

Given the broad nature of consultative medicine, the range of competencies in medical consultation varies little among practice settings. However, the extent and complexity of the role may be determined by the availability of surgical, anesthesia, trauma/critical care, obstetric, psychiatric, and other specialists, including internal medicine subspecialists. Optimal consultative care requires skills that can be adapted to both office practice and a variety of hospital settings, including outpatient and day surgery.

Since medical consultation is practiced at the interface of internal medicine and other specialties, it requires familiarity with those specialties, skill in synthesizing information, and appropriate effective communication with attending and other consulting physicians, dentists, other health care workers, and families.

Common Clinical Presentations

- Evaluation of abnormal result on a routine preoperative test
- Assessment of need for antibiotic prophylaxis for invasive procedure
- Assessment of need for anticoagulation as a prophylactic procedure
- Assessment of need for hemodynamic monitoring during surgery
- Assessment of need for transfer to medical service, including need for critical care monitoring
- Assessment and management of preoperative risk
- Medical problems arising during postoperative recovery
- Medical problems during pregnancy
- Medical problems in psychiatric patients
- Drug reactions and complications

Procedure Skills
> None specific to the discipline

Primary Interpretation of Tests
> • Pre- and postoperative electrocardiography

Ordering and Understanding Tests
> • Noninvasive and invasive assessment of cardiac risk
> • Noninvasive and invasive assessment of venous thromboembolic disease, pre- and postoperatively
> • Pre- and postoperative electrocardiography
> • Pulmonary function testing, including arterial blood gases
> • Routine laboratory data in relationship to planned procedures and surgery

In-depth knowledge of clinical conditions, including principles of management and indications for referral.

CONSULTATIVE MEDICINE

Competency	Priority		Preferred Learning Venues					
			Outpatient			Inpatient	Other	Didactic
	FCIM Task Force	Residency Program	Continuity Clinic	Subspecialty Clinic	Other			
Drug metabolism, reactions, and interactions	1							
Nutritional assessment	1							
Physiologic changes in the elderly	1							
Medical complications of pregnancy	1							
Preoperative evaluation of disease-related risk from surgery	1							
Acute or chronic renal failure	1							
Arrhythmias, conduction disturbances	1							
Chronic obstructive pulmonary disease, asthma	1							
Congestive heart failure	1							
Coronary artery disease	1							
Diabetes mellitus	1							
Electrolyte disorders	1							
Hematologic and clotting disorders	1							
HIV infection	1							
Infectious disease	1							
Obesity	1							
Psychiatric disease	1							
Substance abuse	1							
Thyroid disease	1							

CONSULTATIVE MEDICINE (CONT.)

| Competency | Priority | | Preferred Learning Venues | | | | | |
| | FCIM Task Force | Residency Program | Outpatient | | | Inpatient | | Didactic |
			Continuity Clinic	Subspecialty Clinic	Other	Other	Inpatient	
Preoperative evaluation of disease-related risk from surgery (continued)								
Valvular heart disease	1							
Cerebrovascular or other neurologic disorder	2							
Liver disease	2							
Rheumatologic disorders	2							
Postoperative complications								
Acid-base disorders	1							
Acute renal failure	1							
Adult respiratory distress syndrome	1							
Arrhythmia, cardiac arrest	1							
Atelectasis, pneumonia, aspiration	1							
Chest pain, dyspnea	1							
Delirium	1							
Diabetes	1							
Fever	1							
Hematologic disorders, bleeding	1							
Hypertension, hypotension	1							
Jaundice, liver dysfunction	1							
Postoperative pain	1							
Sepsis, multiorgan failure	1							
Thromboembolic disease	1							

Key: 1 = direct patient responsibility preferred; 2 = any other form of learning that is centered on a patient; 3 = lectures/seminars/reading suffice.

CONSULTATIVE MEDICINE (CONT.)

Competency	Priority		Preferred Learning Venues					
			Outpatient					
	FCIM Task Force	Residency Program	Continuity Clinic	Subspecialty Clinic	Other	Other	Inpatient	Didactic
Postoperative complications (continued)								
Volume, tonicity, or electrolyte disorders	1							
Acute neurologic disease	2							
Gastrointestinal dysfunction	2							
Transfusion reactions	2							
Prevention of complications								
Antibiotic prophylaxis (including for endocarditis)	1							
Postoperative pulmonary complications	1							
Thromboembolism	1							
Reactions to contrast media	2							
Stress-related gastrointestinal mucosal disease	2							

Key: 1 = direct patient responsibility preferred; 2 = any other form of learning that is centered on a patient; 3 = lectures/seminars/reading suffice.

Critical Care Medicine

Overview

Critical care medicine encompasses the diagnosis and treatment of a wide range of clinical problems representing the extreme of human disease. Critically ill patients require intensive care by a coordinated team, including a general internist, subspecialists, and allied health professional staff. Most often, the general internist provides care in coordination with other physicians, especially those trained in critical care. However, in some settings, the general internist may be the primary provider of care and may also serve as a consultant for critically ill patients on surgical services. Therefore, the general internist must have command of a broad range of conditions common among critically ill patients and must be familiar with the technologic procedures and devices used in the intensive care setting. The care of critically ill patients raises many complicated ethical and social issues, and the general internist must be competent in such areas as end-of-life decisions, advance directives, estimating prognosis, and counseling of patients and their families.

Common Clinical Presentations

- Acute abdominal pain
- Acute chest pain
- Acute intoxication
- Acute liver failure
- Acute renal failure
- Altered mental status, coma
- Hypotension, shock
- Life-threatening arrhythmia
- Massive gastrointestinal bleeding
- Massive hemoptysis
- Respiratory distress or failure
- Severe hypertension
- Status epilepticus

Procedure Skills

- Advanced cardiac life support
- Arterial puncture for arterial blood gas
- Bedside pulmonary function
- Mechanical ventilation (basic)
- Placement of arterial and central venous lines
- Placement of nasogastric tube
- Insertion of temporary pacemaker (optional)
- Placement of endotracheal tube (optional)
- Placement of pulmonary artery catheter (optional)

Primary Interpretation of Tests
- Hemodynamic monitoring
- Pulse oximetry
- Telemetry monitoring

Ordering and Understanding Tests
- Bronchoscopy
- Computed tomography, magnetic resonance imaging of chest, abdomen
- Coronary angiography
- Echocardiography
- Electroencephalography

In-depth knowledge of clinical conditions, including principles of management and indications for referral.

CRITICAL CARE MEDICINE

Competency	Priority		Preferred Learning Venues					
			Outpatient				Inpatient	Didactic
	FCIM Task Force	Residency Program	Continuity Clinic	Subspecialty Clinic	Other	Other		
Altitude illness	3							
Burns, smoke inhalation	3							
Cardiac								
Acute myocardial infarction	1							
Acute pericarditis	1							
Aortic dissection	1							
Cardiopulmonary arrest	1							
Congestive heart failure	1							
Dysrhythmias	1							
Hypertensive crisis	1							
Shock	1							
Acute valvular disruption	2							
Myocardial contusion	3							
Decompression illness, air embolism	3							
Near drowning	2							
Drug or alcohol overdose	1							
Drug or alcohol withdrawal	1							

Key: 1 = direct patient responsibility preferred; 2 = any other form of learning that is centered on a patient; 3 = lectures/seminars/reading suffice.

CRITICAL CARE MEDICINE (CONT.)

Competency	Priority		Preferred Learning Venues					
	FCIM Task Force	Residency Program	Outpatient			Other	Inpatient	Didactic
			Continuity Clinic	Subspecialty Clinic	Other			
Endocrine								
Diabetic ketoacidosis, hyperosmolar nonketotic diabetic coma	1							
Adrenal insufficiency	2							
Thyroid storm, myxedema coma	2							
Gastrointestinal								
Acute pancreatitis	1							
Gastrointestinal bleeding	1							
Hepatic failure	1							
Hematologic								
Bleeding disorder	1							
Disseminated intravascular coagulation	1							
Hypothermia, hyperthermia	2							
Infectious								
Nosocomial infection	1							
Septic shock	1							
Management of critical illness								
Multi-organ failure	1							
Prognosis/outcomes	1							
Withdrawal of support	1							

CRITICAL CARE MEDICINE (CONT.)

Competency	Priority		Preferred Learning Venues					
			Outpatient					
	FCIM Task Force	Residency Program	Continuity Clinic	Subspecialty Clinic	Other	Other	Inpatient	Didactic
Neurologic								
Coma	1							
Delirium	1							
Meningitis	1							
Status epilepticus	1							
Stroke	1							
Acute spinal cord injury	2							
Head trauma	2							
Neuromuscular disease with respiratory failure	2							
Nutrition	1							
Pulmonary								
Airway management (intubation, tracheostomy)	1							
Status asthmaticus	1							
Upper airway obstruction	1							
Renal								
Acid-base disturbances	1							
Acute renal failure	1							
Electrolyte imbalance	1							

Key: 1 = direct patient responsibility preferred; 2 = any other form of learning that is centered on a patient; 3 = lectures/seminars/reading suffice.

CRITICAL CARE MEDICINE (CONT.)

Competency	Priority		Preferred Learning Venues					
			Outpatient					
	FCIM Task Force	Residency Program	Continuity Clinic	Subspecialty Clinic	Other	Other	Inpatient	Didactic
Respiratory								
Chronic obstructive pulmonary disease (exacerbated)	1							
Hypercapnia	1							
Hypoxia	1							
Pneumonia	1							
Pneumothorax	1							
Pulmonary embolism	1							
Tuberculosis	1							
Adult respiratory distress syndrome	2							
Hemoptysis	2							
Chest trauma	3							

Key: 1 = direct patient responsibility preferred; 2 = any other form of learning that is centered on a patient; 3 = lectures/seminars/reading suffice.

Emergency Medicine

Overview

Emergency medicine involves the evaluation and care of acute illness and injuries that require intervention within a limited time span. It is defined by a time interval rather than by a particular organ. Some conditions may be encountered in office practice, others in acute care settings. Regardless of the setting, the general internist should be able to manage common emergency conditions and provide consultation and management for a variety of acute serious illnesses.

The range of competencies expected of a general internist will depend on the availability of emergency physicians and other specialists in the community.

Common Clinical Presentations

- Abdominal pain
- Acute loss of vision
- Cardiac arrest
- Cardiac dysrhythmias
- Chest pain
- Coma, altered mental status
- Dehydration
- Diarrhea
- Dyspnea
- Gastrointestinal bleeding
- Headache
- Hemoptysis
- Hip fracture
- Leg swelling
- Musculoskeletal trauma
- Palpitations
- Severe hypertension
- Shock
- Syncope
- Vaginal bleeding
- Volume depletion
- Vomiting
- Wheezing

Procedure Skills
- Advanced cardiac life support
- Arthrocentesis
- Fluorescent staining of cornea
- Mask ventilation to maintain airway
- Needle decompression of tension pneumothorax
- Placement of nasogastric tube
- Insertion of temporary pacemaker (optional)
- Pericardiocentesis (optional)
- Suturing of laceration (optional)

Ordering and Understanding Tests
- Aortography
- Computed tomography of head, chest, abdomen
- Echocardiography
- Noninvasive vascular studies
- Pulmonary angiography
- Toxicology studies
- Ultrasound of abdomen, pelvis
- Ventilation/perfusion scans of the lungs

In-depth knowledge of clinical conditions, including principles of management and indications for referral.

EMERGENCY MEDICINE

Competency	Priority		Preferred Learning Venues					
			Outpatient			Other	Inpatient	Didactic
	FCIM Task Force	Residency Program	Continuity Clinic	Subspecialty Clinic	Other			
Cardiovascular								
Acute or chronic congestive heart failure	1							
Arrhythmias	1							
Cardiopulmonary arrest	1							
Chest pain, stable and unstable angina, myocardial infarction	1							
Hypertension, hypertensive emergencies	1							
Shock	1							
Syncope	1							
Unstable thoracic or abdominal aortic aneurysms	2							
Dermatologic								
Rash	1							
Cutaneous ulcers	2							
Domestic violence	1							
Endocrine								
Diabetes mellitus, hypo-glycemia, hyperglycemia, diabetic ketoacidosis	1							
Acute complications of hyper-thyroidism, hypothyroidism	2							
Addisonian crisis	2							

Key: 1 = direct patient responsibility preferred; 2 = any other form of learning that is centered on a patient; 3 = lectures/seminars/reading suffice.

EMERGENCY MEDICINE (CONT.)

Competency	Priority		Preferred Learning Venues					
			Outpatient				Inpatient	Didactic
	FCIM Task Force	Residency Program	Continuity Clinic	Subspecialty Clinic	Other	Other		
Gastroenterologic								
Acute abdomen	1							
Acute diarrhea	1							
Acute liver failure	1							
Acute pancreatitis	1							
Ascites	1							
Bleeding	1							
Gallstones, cholecystitis	1							
Bowel obstruction	2							
Hematologic								
Acute complications of sickle cell disease	1							
Anemia, leukopenia, thrombocytopenia	2							
Easy bruising, purpura, ecchymosis	2							
Polycythemia, leukocytosis, thrombocytosis	3							
Hyperthermia, hypothermia	2							

EMERGENCY MEDICINE (CONT.)

Competency	Priority		Preferred Learning Venues					
			Outpatient			Inpatient	Didactic	
	FCIM Task Force	Residency Program	Continuity Clinic	Subspecialty Clinic	Other	Other		
Infections								
Active tuberculosis	1							
Herpes zoster infection	1							
HIV infection (including *Infectious complications*)	1							
Meningitis	1							
Otitis externa media	1							
Pharyngitis	1							
Pneumonia, bronchitis	1							
Prostatitis, urethritis, epididymitis	1							
Sepsis	1							
Sexually transmitted diseases	1							
Sinusitis	1							
Upper respiratory infection	1							
Urinary tract infection, pyelonephritis	1							
Viral hepatitis	1							
Herpes simplex infection	2							
Encephalitis	3							

Key: 1 = direct patient responsibility preferred; 2 = any other form of learning that is centered on a patient; 3 = lectures/seminars/reading suffice.

EMERGENCY MEDICINE (CONT.)

Competency	Priority		Preferred Learning Venues					
				Outpatient			Inpatient	Didactic
	FCIM Task Force	Residency Program	Continuity Clinic	Subspecialty Clinic	Other	Other		
Neurologic								
Coma	1							
Head trauma	1							
Headache	1							
Seizure	1							
Transient ischemic attack, stroke, subarachnoid hemorrhage	1							
Ophthalmologic								
Red eye	1							
Acute loss of vision	2							
Otolaryngologic								
Epistaxis	1							
Vertigo	1							
Overdose, poisoning	1							
Pulmonary								
Acute respiratory failure	1							
Asthma	1							
Chronic obstructive pulmonary disease	1							
Pneumothorax	1							
Pulmonary embolism, deep venous thrombosis, phlebitis	1							
Severe airway obstruction	1							

EMERGENCY MEDICINE (CONT.)

| Competency | Priority | | Preferred Learning Venues | | | | | | |
	FCIM Task Force	Residency Program	Continuity Clinic	Subspecialty Clinic	Other	Other	Inpatient	Didactic
				Outpatient				
Renal								
Acute renal failure, chronic renal insufficiency	1							
Electrolyte, acid-base disorders	1							
Renal colic, kidney stones	1							
Rheumatologic								
Acute arthritis (including gout)	1							
Back pain	1							
Sexual abuse	1							

Key: 1 = direct patient responsibility preferred; **2** = any other form of learning that is centered on a patient; **3** = lectures/seminars/reading suffice.

THE CLINICAL COMPETENCIES

Population-Specific Clinical Competencies

- Adolescent Medicine

- Geriatrics

- Substance Abuse

- Women's Health and Office Gynecology

Adolescent Medicine

Overview

Adolescent medicine is a core aspect of general internal medicine practice. It differs from other subspecialties in that diagnosis is usually more complicated than treatment: The challenge is in the evaluation of nonspecific complaints. Few diseases are specific to adolescents. General internists should be familiar with chronic childhood diseases and should be alert to early signs and symptoms of diseases seen in adults. Adolescent medicine includes a large behavioral component. Some general internists develop a special expertise and focus their practice in adolescent medicine.

Common Clinical Presentations
- Abdominal pain (recurring)
- Amenorrhea
- Delayed development
- Depression
- Fatigue
- Headache
- Irregular vaginal bleeding
- Male breast swelling
- Poor or altered school performance (including truancy)
- Risk-taking behavior
- Surveillance after treatment of malignancy in childhood
- Weight loss or gain

Procedure Skills
- First pelvic examination
- Tanner staging (optional)

Primary Interpretation of Tests
- Height/weight growth charts (optional)

Ordering and Understanding Tests
- Wrist radiography (to determine bone age) (optional)

In-depth knowledge of clinical conditions, including principles of management and indications for referral.

ADOLESCENT MEDICINE

| Competency | Priority | | Preferred Learning Venues | | | | | |
| | | | Outpatient | | | Inpatient | Other | Didactic |
	FCIM Task Force	Residency Program	Continuity Clinic	Subspecialty Clinic	Other			
Acne	1							
Amenorrhea (primary and secondary)	1							
Behavior risks (assessment and counseling)								
Cigarette smoking	1							
HIV	1							
Reckless behavior	1							
Self-image issues	1							
Sexual activity (unprotected)	1							
Substance abuse	1							
Behavioral management of chronic disease	1							
Crohn's disease	2							
Delayed development	2							
Depression	1							
Domestic violence	1							
Eating disorders								
Anorexia nervosa	1							
Bulimia nervosa	1							
Obesity/hyperphagia	2							

ADOLESCENT MEDICINE (CONT.)

Competency	Priority		Preferred Learning Venues					
	FCIM Task Force	Residency Program	Outpatient			Inpatient	Didactic
			Continuity Clinic	Subspecialty Clinic	Other	Other		
Insulin-dependent diabetes	1							
Learning disabilities	3							
Migraine headache	1							
Scoliosis	2							
Sexually transmitted diseases	1							
Societal violence	1							
Sports injuries	1							

Key: 1 = direct patient responsibility preferred; 2 = any other form of learning that is centered on a patient; 3 = lectures/seminars/reading suffice.

Geriatrics

Overview

Competency in clinical geriatrics involves recognizing the difference in presentation of disease and the importance of maintaining functional independence in elderly patients. With increasing age, presentations of disease become less classic and are often muted, and timely recognition requires attentiveness to subtle signs. Appropriate management requires a balance of patient observation, judicious diagnostic intervention, and acceptance of limits as defined by the patient. Effective management of problems may be complex and may necessitate an interdisciplinary approach that takes social support into account. Medical and psychological problems, acute and chronic, frequently coexist.

Many competencies of geriatrics are included within lists for other disciplines. They are repeated here to reflect the unique set of skills required to manage specific problems when they occur in the elderly.

Common Clinical Presentations

- Change in affect (depression, mania)
- Change in cognition (chronic, subacute, acute)
- Elder mistreatment
- Failure to thrive, frailty
- Falls, gait disorders
- Fecal obstipation or incontinence
- Immobility
- Inability to feed or take care of oneself
- Inadequate home support
- Loss of hearing
- Loss of vision
- Neurobehavioral disorders (agitation, psychosis, anxiety)
- Pain
- Postural instability
- Pressure sores
- Sleep disorders
- Syncope, dizziness
- Urinary retention or incontinence
- Weight loss

Procedure Skills
- Cognitive assessment
- Evaluation of decision-making capacity
- Functional assessment
- Gait assessment
- Home safety assessment
- Motor vehicle driving assessment
- Needs assessment on hospital discharge, including rehabilitation
- Rectal disimpaction

Primary Interpretation of Tests
- Nutrition screening
- Voiding record

Ordering and Understanding Tests
- Urodynamic testing, cystometry
- Measurement of intraocular pressure
- Audiology
- Neuropsychiatric testing
- Videofluoroscopy for swallowing problems
- Noninvasive tests of peripheral arteries
- Biopsy of temporal artery

In-depth knowledge of clinical conditions, including principles of management and indications for referral.

GERIATRICS

| Competency | Priority | | Preferred Learning Venues | | | | | |
| | FCIM Task Force | Residency Program | Outpatient | | | Other | Inpatient | Didactic |
			Continuity Clinic	Subspecialty Clinic	Other			
Accident risk								
Falls	1							
Gait disorders	1							
Poor safety awareness	1							
Cardiovascular								
Angina/myocardial infarction	1							
Congestive heart failure	1							
Hypertension	1							
Lower-extremity edema	1							
Orthostatic hypotension	1							
Abdominal aneurysm	2							
Death and dying	1							
Elder mistreatment	1							
Endocrine/metabolic								
Dehydration	1							
Non–insulin-dependent and insulin-dependent diabetes	1							
Disorders of temperature regulation	2							
Thyroid disorder								
Hyperthyroid	2							
Hypothyroid	2							
Sick euthyroid	2							

GERIATRICS (CONT.)

Competency	Priority		Preferred Learning Venues					
			Outpatient			Inpatient	Other	Didactic
	FCIM Task Force	Residency Program	Continuity Clinic	Subspecialty Clinic	Other			
Ethical issues (advance directives, health care proxy, unrealistic expectations of family and patient)	1							
Failure to thrive	1							
Gastroenterologic								
Constipation, obstipation	1							
Fecal incontinence	1							
Peptic ulcer disease	1							
Swallowing disorders	1							
Ischemic bowel	2							
Hematologic								
Anemia	1							
Multiple myeloma	1							
Iatrogenic disease								
Adverse drug reactions	1							
Nosocomial complications	1							
Polypharmacy, drug interactions	1							
Procedure complications	2							
Neurologic								
Carotid artery disease	1							
Parkinson's disease	1							
Stroke	1							
Transient ischemic attack	1							

Key: 1 = direct patient responsibility preferred; 2 = any other form of learning that is centered on a patient; 3 = lectures/seminars/reading suffice.

GERIATRICS (CONT.)

Competency	Priority		Preferred Learning Venues					
	FCIM Task Force	Residency Program	Outpatient				Inpatient	Didactic
			Continuity Clinic	Subspecialty Clinic	Other	Other		
Nutrition								
Aspiration	1							
Aspiration pneumonia	1							
Feeding disorders	1							
Malnutrition	1							
Oral health problems	2							
Pain control	1							
Pneumonia	1							
Psychiatric								
Alcoholism, drug abuse	1							
Delirium	1							
Dementia	1							
Depression	1							
Neurobehavioral disorders	1							
Social isolation	1							
Late-onset psychotic disorders	2							
Renal/Urologic								
Prostate disease	1							
Sexual dysfunction	1							
Urinary incontinence	1							
Urinary retention	1							
Urinary tract infection	1							

GERIATRICS (CONT.)

Competency	Priority		Preferred Learning Venues					
			Outpatient			Inpatient	Other	Didactic
	FCIM Task Force	Residency Program	Continuity Clinic	Subspecialty Clinic	Other			
Rheumatologic/Musculoskeletal								
Contractures	1							
Crystal diseases (gout, pseudogout)	1							
Deconditioning	1							
Degenerative joint disease	1							
Fractures								
Hip	1							
Vertebral compression fracture	1							
Wrist (Colles')	2							
Other	3							
Immobility	1							
Low-back pain	1							
Osteoporosis	1							
Pressure ulcers	1							
Giant cell arteritis	2							
Polymyalgia rheumatica	2							
Sensory impairment								
Hearing								
Cerumen impaction	1							
Presbycusis	1							
Meniere's disease	3							
Peripheral neuropathy	1							

Key: 1 = direct patient responsibility preferred; 2 = any other form of learning that is centered on a patient; 3 = lectures/seminars/reading suffice.

GERIATRICS (CONT.)

Competency	Priority		Preferred Learning Venues					
	FCIM Task Force	Residency Program	Continuity Clinic	Subspecialty Clinic	Other	Other	Inpatient	Didactic
			Outpatient					
Vision								
Cataracts	1							
Glaucoma	1							
Macular degeneration	1							
Vestibular disorders	2							
Skin cancer	1							
Sleep disorders	1							
Syncope	1							
Tuberculosis	2							

Key: 1 = direct patient responsibility preferred; 2 = any other form of learning that is centered on a patient; 3 = lectures/seminars/reading suffice.

Substance Abuse

Overview

The harmful use of and addiction to alcohol and other drugs—including prescription drugs—is one of this nation's major and most costly health problems. Excluding nicotine, alcohol and other drug problems are present in 10% to 20% of ambulatory patients and in 25% to 50% of general hospital patients. Since over 20% of U.S. adults are regular cigarette smokers, nicotine addiction adds measurably to the already high prevalence. Despite its high prevalence, physicians (and sometimes patients themselves) often fail to recognize a substance abuse problem. Also, because of the stigma attached to substance abuse, people with this problem may not reveal it to their physician. Making this diagnosis is a high priority since substance abuse and dependence cause numerous medical problems, may masquerade as other psychiatric diagnoses, and may complicate ongoing therapeutic management of other diseases. The primary care physician is the first line of defense in recognizing and treating disorders of substance abuse and addiction.

Common Clinical Presentations

- Repeated injury
- Systolic hypertension (alcohol)
- Chronic insomnia
- Chronic pain without an evident diagnosis
- Fatigue, memory impairment
- Panic or anxiety attacks
- Depression secondary to ETOH/sedative drugs
- Weight loss (stimulant abuse, AIDS)
- HIV+/AIDS
- Substance-abusing health professional

Manifestations of Alcohol/Sedative Withdrawal

- Agitation
- Insomnia
- Seizures
- Delirium
- Hallucinations

Manifestations of Opioid Withdrawal

- Insomnia
- Profuse diaphoresis
- Lacrimation, rhinorrhea
- Piloerection (goose flesh)
- Shallow breathing; respiratory arrest

Manifestations of Opioid Intoxication
- Pinpoint pupils
- Clammy skin
- Needle tracks
- Somnolence, confusion

Cocaine or Amphetamine Intoxication
- Agitation
- Dilated pupils
- Rapid mood swings
- Aggressive behavior

Procedure Skills (Including Essential Clinical Skills)
- Interview in order to screen for tobacco, alcohol, and other drug use and any problems related to their consumption
- Counseling and management of substance abuse and alcohol abuse, including appropriate use of referrals
- Counseling intravenous drug users about HIV risk
- Skill in presenting a diagnosis of addiction and initiating an appropriate referral for specialized care

Primary Interpretation of Tests
- Drug screening via blood and urine tests
- Blood and breath alcohol tests

Ordering and Understanding Tests
- Blood and breath alcohol levels
- Urine tests for drugs
- HIV, hepatitis
- Mean corpuscular red blood cell volume

In-depth knowledge of clinical conditions, including principles of management and indications for referral.

SUBSTANCE ABUSE

Competency	Priority		Preferred Learning Venues					
			Outpatient				Inpatient	Didactic
	FCIM Task Force	Residency Program	Continuity Clinic	Subspecialty Clinic	Other	Other		
Alcohol								
Rehabilitation	1							
Withdrawal syndrome	1							
Cocaine								
Acute toxicity	1							
Chronic abuse	2							
High-risk behavior for HIV	1							
LSD and PCP intoxication	3							
Marijuana intoxication	3							
Opioid withdrawal syndrome	2							
Pain								
Acute	1							
Chronic	1							
Sedative/hypnotic addiction	2							
Tobacco cessation	1							

Key: 1 = direct patient responsibility preferred; 2 = any other form of learning that is centered on a patient; 3 = didactic learning suffices.

Women's Health and Office Gynecology

Overview

Women's health embraces the spectrum of health-related issues for women, from screening and prevention to management of acute and chronic illness. Its knowledge base focuses on the specific risk factors, physiologic variables, and therapeutic options that apply to women across the life cycle. Its knowledge base overlaps with and draws from the fields of gynecology, endocrinology, nutrition, psychiatry, and general internal medicine. Some general internists focus their practice on women's health issues, but all general internists should be well informed and competent in this area.

Women's health addresses conditions that are unique to, more common in, or more serious in women or that have manifestations, risk factors, or interventions that are different in women. Conditions affecting women, in which sex- and gender-based differences are not known, are listed under other categories in this document. In this section, the emphasis is on diseases specific to or more prevalent in women.

Common Clinical Presentations

- Abnormal menstruation, vaginal bleeding
- Abnormal Papanicolaou smear
- Bladder pain
- Breast symptoms (lump, tenderness, nipple discharge)
- Contraception, request for
- Cystocele, rectocele, enterocele, uterine prolapse
- Dyspareunia
- Galactorrhea, nipple discharge
- Genital warts and ulcers
- Hirsutism
- Incest
- Incontinence (urinary and fecal)
- Infertility
- Life-phase issues
- Menopausal symptoms
- Pelvic mass
- Pelvic pain
- Physical/emotional abuse
- Post-trauma stress disorder
- Preconception and postconception counseling, request for
- Pregnancy
- Premenstrual syndrome
- Rape, symptoms of violence and assault
- Sexuality issues
- Vaginal symptoms (discharge, itching, odor, dryness)
- Varicose veins, venous disease

Procedure Skills

- Counseling about cosmetic/reconstructive surgery
- Crisis counseling/psychosocial counseling
- Fitting of diaphragm
- Rape protocol
- Removal of foreign body from vagina
- Colposcopy (optional)
- Endometrial biopsy (optional)
- Insertion and removal of intrauterine device (optional)
- Office urodynamics (optional)
- Administration of contraceptives
- Administration of hormone replacement therapy

Primary Interpretation of Tests

- Urine pregnancy test
- Pelvic ultrasound

Ordering and Understanding Tests

- Aspiration of breast mass
- Bladder function tests
- Bone densitometry
- *Chlamydia* culture
- Colposcopy and biopsy
- Computed tomography of the abdomen, pelvis
- Dilatation and curettage
- Endometrial biopsy
- Fertility studies
- Incision and drainage of breast abscess
- Laparoscopy
- Mammography
- Papanicolaou pathology report
- Sex hormone assays

In-depth knowledge of clinical conditions, including principles of management and indications for referral.

WOMEN'S HEALTH AND OFFICE GYNECOLOGY

Competency	Priority		Preferred Learning Venues					
			Outpatient					
	FCIM Task Force	Residency Program	Continuity Clinic	Subspecialty Clinic	Other	Other	Inpatient	Didactic
Breast disease								
Breast cancer	1							
Breast mass	1							
Fibrocystic disease	2							
Breast reconstruction, augmentation, or reduction	3							
Counseling								
Breast-feeding	1							
Eating disorders	1							
Physical/emotional abuse	1							
Pregnancy	1							
Sexual assault	1							
Gynecology disorders								
Abnormal Papanicolaou smear	1							
Cervical cancer	1							
Endometriosis	1							
Fibroids	1							
Genital herpes	1							
Pelvic inflammatory disease	1							
Vaginitis	1							
Ovarian cyst	2							
Infertility	3							

WOMEN'S HEALTH AND OFFICE GYNECOLOGY (CONT.)

Competency	Priority		Preferred Learning Venues					
			Outpatient			Other	Inpatient	Didactic
	FCIM Task Force	Residency Program	Continuity Clinic	Subspecialty Clinic	Other			
Normal pregnancy								
Nutrition	2							
Postpartum depression	2							
Abnormal pregnancy								
Emotional impact of abortion/miscarriage	2							
Threatened/spontaneous abortion	2							
Ectopic pregnancy	3							
Menstrual								
Amenorrhea (primary, secondary)	1							
Dysmenorrhea	1							
Hormone replacement therapy	1							
Menopause	1							
Premenstrual syndrome	1							
Unexplained vaginal bleeding	1							
Osteoporosis	1							
Pregnancy								
Medical complications	1							
Normal physiology	1							

Key: 1 = direct patient responsibility preferred; 2 = any other form of learning that is centered on a patient; 3 = lectures/seminars/reading suffice.

WOMEN'S HEALTH AND OFFICE GYNECOLOGY (CONT.)

Competency	Priority		Preferred Learning Venues					
			Outpatient			Inpatient	Didactic
	FCIM Task Force	Residency Program	Continuity Clinic	Subspecialty Clinic	Other	Other		
Sex-related								
Contraception	1							
Sexual dysfunction	1							
Sexually transmitted diseases	1							
Sexuality over the life cycle	2							
Sexual preference and identity	3							
Urinary disorder								
Incontinence	1							
Interstitial cystitis	2							

Key: 1 = direct patient responsibility preferred; 2 = any other form of learning that is centered on a patient; 3 = lectures/seminars/reading suffice.

CHAPTER 7

THE LEARNING EXPERIENCE: ROTATIONS AND VENUES

Novice flyers become professional pilots by flying airplanes, and journeyman carvers become master craftsmen by working at the bench. Similarly, medical students and residents learn to become doctors by treating patients in the hospital and, more recently, in the office and other settings.

The actual practice of medicine is multidimensional and provides the most effective form of learning. In medical education, this practice historically has evolved from apprenticeship to hospital-based clerkship. However, since medical care has changed, these traditional experiences may fail to represent the real world of practice. For those reasons, medical educators must scrutinize all educational experiences carefully, gauging each by the value it provides.

This curricular resource document considers all formal resident time assignments, such as inpatient rotations and ambulatory clinics, to be experiences, or venues, with specific educational objectives. The place of each venue in the curriculum depends upon the competencies it conveys and the opportunities it offers for learning and acculturation.

The descriptions of the venues of learning, which appear in this section, serve two purposes. The first is to illustrate how the venues provide access to the competencies in the curriculum. The second purpose is to identify the critical determinants of learning within each venue: resident responsibility, faculty-resident interactions, patient selection, and resources for learning.

The Learning Venues

Inpatient Rotations

The care of hospitalized patients provides the opportunity for residents to learn diagnostic and management skills in a condensed, efficient way. This venue has had a century-long tradition and, as the keystone of residency training, is well known to medical educators and trainees alike. Nonetheless, it is appropriate to examine this venue in the context of curricular objectives.

The ideal inpatient ward experience should allow the resident to refine history and physical examination skills, develop experience in the selection of diagnostic tests, and learn to manage a wide variety of diseases. Although reduced lengths of hospital stay may adversely impact learning opportunities on inpatient wards, a major advantage of the hospital-based setting is the rapid feedback that residents

179

frequently receive after they order diagnostic tests or begin new treatments. Ideally, residents have the chance while on inpatient wards to make a diagnosis, select a treatment, and see the initial results of the prescribed therapy.

During hospital rotations, residents acquire intensive experience working with other health care personnel, including nurses, social workers, pharmacists, ward clerks, residents from other specialties, and attending physicians from other disciplines. Residents on hospital-based rotations learn to interact with patients and families in the acute care setting; they also learn the communications skills needed for dealing with referring physicians and other health care personnel.

Inpatient rotations have traditionally been scheduled throughout the 3 years of residency. This approach provides residents with increasing supervisory and teaching responsibility as they gain clinical experience. Typically, while on the inpatient rotations, residents have one-half day of "continuity clinic" but spend the remainder of their time dedicated to care of hospitalized patients. Other models of inpatient experiences may offer advantages. Some programs have moved to a "50% ambulatory residency" that contains as few as 8 months of inpatient (non–intensive care unit [ICU]) rotations over the course of 3 years of training. Another model of inpatient experience is to mix the care of inpatients with daily experience in an ambulatory clinic. Few programs currently use this model, but it has the advantage of providing training experience similar to the actual practice of internal medicine.

Ideal inpatient experiences have dedicated teaching space, effective hospital systems for ancillary support, and a diverse patient population. The most effective teaching site is the general medical service on which there is a mix of patients with diverse medical problems. Subspecialty-oriented inpatient services (for example, cardiology or oncology) can also be effective venues for resident education if this experience is directed at acquiring specific competencies.

Many sources contribute to the educational experience in the inpatient service. Traditional inpatient teams include one or more interns supervised by a second- or third-year resident under the overall supervision of an attending physician. This team structure permits residents to have "graded responsibility" for decisions regarding patient care. The attending physician should be directly involved with patient care on a daily basis. All teaching rounds should focus on the patient and should include bedside teaching of history and physical examination. Teaching rounds should also provide an opportunity to refine case presentation skills, discuss appropriate selection of diagnostic tests and management strategies, review pathophysiology, and teach psychosocial issues related to patient care. Patient-oriented teaching rounds should be supplemented by didactic presentations and conferences designed to ensure comprehensive coverage of a range of diseases appropriate for internal medicine training.

The rapidly changing dynamics of the inpatient rotation provide constant educational challenges. Before the era of cost containment, the inpatient service was an efficient and effective learning environment because virtually all patients were hospitalized until they recovered completely. This practice allowed the resident to participate in the complete continuum of diagnosis and treatment. This leisurely environment no longer exists. Now patients enter the hospital for specific therapy after having been diagnosed as an outpatient and may be discharged before the outcomes of therapy are certain. Thus, it is increasingly difficult to provide residents with the experience of making a diagnosis, selecting therapy, and observing the results of the prescribed therapy.

Because the stay in the hospital is often very brief now, inpatient rotations may provide only a glimpse of the evolving course of the patient's illness. This reality poses formidable educational challenges. The primary purpose of the inpatient rotation is to gain experience with acute illness. Therefore, the inpatient service should be organized to optimize this experience and minimize exposure to routine short-stay patients. A second challenge is teaching residents the important new skill of managing the seamless transition of patient care from the hospital to the ambulatory setting. The resident must coordinate health care and social services during hospitalization so that the patient can use these services effectively after discharge. The resident must communicate with consultants and the patient's regular physician. Acquiring this skill and learning how to use resources prudently must form the foundation of experience on the inpatient service.

Critical Care Medicine

The vast majority of acute care hospitals in the United States have at least one ICU, and ICU beds make up 5% to 10% of all acute care beds. In these facilities, seriously ill patients receive sophisticated monitoring and often advanced life support. Many common but life-threatening syndromes, such as adult respiratory distress syndrome and septic shock, are always treated in the ICU and require coordinated physician and nursing teamwork. Internists are usually key members of these teams and may serve a variety of roles, ranging from primary care provider to ICU director. Therefore, all internists should have training and experience in the diagnosis and management of patients in the critical care setting.

Since critical care is physically and emotionally taxing, the length of the ICU rotation should not exceed 4 weeks. Housestaff will learn the most from intensive care training if they experience it when they are at different levels of clinical sophistication and self-confidence. Therefore, ideally, critical care rotations will occur in 2 or more years of the 3-year residency.

Critical care training should occur in a distinct intensive care unit with a fully dedicated nursing staff and ICU director. The ICU team comprises a wide array of health care professionals, including consultants, primary care physicians, intensivists, nurses, social workers, respiratory therapists, and others. Preferably, the ICU experience occurs on a general medical unit, but a mixed medical-surgical unit is a reasonable alternative. Many hospitals also have a separate cardiac care unit (CCU). The CCU is usually excellent for advanced cardiology training but may not have the depth or breadth of other general medical intensive care problems to provide sufficient experience for the resident in training. A CCU experience is not the same as that provided by a general medical ICU.

The organization of critical care practice varies among institutions. In larger hospitals with several ICUs, the staff are full-time critical care physicians. In smaller hospitals, primary care physicians and consulting subspecialists collaborate in providing critical care. For trainees, these different practice patterns may complicate the approach to teaching. As with emergency medicine, intensive care training is a total-immersion experience that should be free from other inpatient service responsibilities. Therefore, residents should be assigned full-time to the ICU rotation and work in one or more housestaff teams. With this arrangement, they can focus their full attention on the care of critically ill patients, the learning of curricular topics in critical care, and first-hand experience with the ICU health care professional team.

The teaching of critical care should be organized and led by experienced intensivists. Whether or not the critical care faculty are the physicians-of-record for the critically ill patients assigned to the resident, they should have the special training and experience in critical care to provide clinical guidance and perspective as well as formal teaching on key curricular topics.

Like many aspects of medical practice, the ebb and flow of clinical material is unpredictable. However, because of the brief but intense nature of the ICU rotation, the faculty should make every reasonable effort to optimize the diversity of the resident's experience. Therefore, it is important to avoid an unbalanced experience—such as many patients admitted just for routine monitoring or, at the other extreme, an experience composed solely of patients with multi-organ failure. Simple corrective steps, such as redistributing residents' patients and discontinuing resident coverage of routinely monitored beds, will avoid an imbalanced experience in which the resident misses opportunities to acquire needed intensive care competencies.

All residents should have a formal orientation to the ICU before beginning their rotation. This orientation should, when necessary, review topics that the resident may have to use under urgent circumstance soon after starting the rotation. Examples could include cardiopulmonary resuscitation, simple procedures, common ICU medications, ICU order sets, and others. The use of such audiovisual aids as videotapes or computer simulation can facilitate learning. A second goal of orientation is to introduce the resident to the personnel, administrative procedures, and culture of the ICU health care team. The final goal of orientation is to explain the educational objectives of the rotation and how they will be achieved through rounds, lectures, educational materials, and other means.

An important goal of the critical care rotation is to cover the key topics with which every internist should be familiar. Some of these topics can be covered in the context of discussing patients currently in the ICU. However, this approach is not likely to cover all the important curricular topics. Therefore, all ICU rotations should provide the means to cover core ICU material adequately. Creative approaches include lectures and demonstrations, video materials, computer simulation, a printed syllabus, and a bibliography.

Emergency Medicine

Internists must often evaluate and manage patients with acute, serious illness. Some internists staff emergency rooms, and all internists must be skilled in the evaluation, stabilization, and triage of patients presenting as emergencies. Rotations in the emergency room (ER) are the best way to gain this experience.

For many patients, the emergency room is the principal interface with the hospital. Patients with acute medical, surgical, toxicologic, traumatic, and psychiatric problems populate hospital emergency rooms. In addition, many patients who might more appropriately receive care in facilities designed for less urgent problems use the emergency room as a point of entry to the health care system for episodic care. Internal medicine residents need experience dealing with the full spectrum of patients and situations in the hospital emergency room.

During the emergency medicine rotation, residents should have direct contact experience in the initial evaluation and stabilization of patients who are acutely ill because of cardiopulmonary diseases, gastrointestinal bleeding, cerebrovascular diseases, septic shock, and shock from other causes, including trauma. Equally important is learning how to distinguish patients who require acute hospitalization from those who can be treated and discharged. The emergency medicine rotation also provides a venue in which medicine residents learn to work with surgeons in stabilizing patients with acute surgical problems.

Residents should gain considerable experience in performing procedures needed for the diagnosis and management of acute medical and surgical diseases, including those that might be considered urgent care. Examples include simple laceration repair and evaluation of acute musculoskeletal injury. Residents should be ACLS-certified prior to beginning emergency medicine rotations and should acquire further practical experience in cardiopulmonary resuscitation during the rotation.

As in all other venues, attending physicians should directly supervise residents in emergency medicine rotations. In some settings, a single resident may work directly with an attending physician. In other settings, second- and third-year residents may directly supervise interns, under the overall supervision of an attending physician. Since the attending physician must be involved directly in the care of each patient, the majority of teaching will be directly patient-oriented. Residents should also gain experience in post-emergency care of patients, whether in the hospital or after discharge. This experience allows them to place the acute evaluation and therapy in the emergency room in the context of overall patient care.

The emergency room experience lends itself to teaching certain curricular goals in assessing and treating acutely ill patients, and most program directors will assign a long list of competencies to the emergency room rotation. Most residents will have difficulty acquiring all the competencies assigned to this rotation through their own care experience. Formats such as lectures, videos, and computer-based instruction provide access to a wide range of topics and complement the experiences acquired in direct patient care.

Continuity Practice Experience

A well-run ambulatory practice for residents should closely duplicate the office practice of internal medicine. In addition to the specific clinical knowledge provided by the medical problems of the patients, the continuity clinic experience teaches residents to take responsibility for patients and relate to them as individuals. Residents learn to recognize medical problems that are in a relatively early stage. They can observe the natural history of illness and address treatable aspects of the patient's illness. Trainees can gain experience as a member of the health care team working closely with other health care professionals.

While there are no well-established scheduling guidelines, the commitment of time to the continuity practice experience should be substantial because most general internal medicine is now grounded in office practice. Since skills develop with experience, the amount of time residents spend in the continuity practice may be a limiting factor in their growth as primary care physicians. Many programs are re-evaluating the amount of time that their residents will spend in the continuity practice experience.

The continuity practice experience should provide a clinical site that is well furnished, clean, and comfortable, with adequate staff for scheduling, maintaining records, retrieving test results, and all the other functions necessary for a well-run practice. Within the clinic setting, teaching space should be well appointed and comfortable. Books, computers, and electronic text retrieval systems should be available, along with systems for laboratory test results retrieval. Residents should have adequate secretarial and nursing assistance. Systems for providing urgent care and off-hours care should be in place.

Programs may choose from one of two models of supervision and instruction. Attending faculty can supervise one or two residents while seeing some patients themselves, or they may schedule no personal patients while supervising a larger number of residents. Each model has its advantages. In neither should residents have to wait more than a few minutes to present cases, nor should the amount of time available for each case discussion average less than 5 minutes. If each resident sees six patients per session, he or she will require at least 30 minutes of individualized instruction, limiting a preceptor who is not seeing his or her own patients to a maximum of six residents in a session. Recent HCFA regulations governing teaching physicians who are providing supervision in primary care settings are an important consideration in determining staffing ratios. Continuity practice preceptors should ideally always work with the same residents and their patient panels.

The concept of team care is as important in continuity clinic as in inpatient rotations. The outpatient continuity practice team generally includes residents, mid-level practitioners, and attending physicians, as well as nurses and appointment secretaries. The organization must provide continuous access to care for patients whose primary resident may be practicing only 1 or 2 half-days per week. Many programs have extended the team concept into firms, linking outpatient and inpatient assignments, so that an identifiable group of house officers care for a prescribed panel of patients in both settings. Communication systems are vital to the success of the team structure by ensuring that clinical information is available wherever the patient is seen and by keeping the patient's primary resident informed.

Residents require formal instruction in outpatient medicine. This instruction should focus on the common ambulatory problems as well as on prevention, screening, behavioral modification, and other important subjects. Several formats are appropriate. Programs may present these topics as part of an ongoing weekly lecture series for all housestaff, as decentralized pre- or post-clinic conferences, or within ambulatory block rotations. Most programs will use all these options. These presentations should be cohesive, organized around a predetermined syllabus, keyed to the competencies of internal medicine, and complementary to other didactic programs.

Access to patients may become an increasing challenge for ambulatory education programs. In the past, clinics staffed by residents attracted disadvantaged patients whose publicly supported health insurance was unattractive to private practitioners. However, in the current era of managed care, these same patients offer favorable reimbursement to private practices, which may entice patients away from the resident clinics. This influence of managed care offers both a challenge and an educational opportunity. The challenge is to structure the continuity clinic so that it remains both desirable to patients and successful in a competitive managed care market. Continuity experience organized in this way will offer residents excellent preparation for practice in the world of managed care. Educational programs that fail to adapt to managed care will become irrelevant to patients, insurers, and ultimately to trainees.

Program directors should pay particular attention to the resident's patient population. Currently, some teaching clinics serve only indigent patients, military veterans, or similarly selected populations. Program directors should make every effort to diversify the resident's exposure, which may require community practice assignments to complement hospital-based clinics. Many programs have required residents to keep a log of their clinic patients and their problems. By paying attention to a resident's accumulated experience, the clinic residency director can distribute patients to residents in a way that maximizes each resident's exposure to a broad array of medical problems and assures them the opportunity to acquire the competencies listed in Chapters 5 and 6 of this book.

Inpatient General Medicine Consult Service

A traditional role for the internist has been to serve as a hospital consultant, particularly on surgical services. Consequently, training programs have usually included a block rotation during which the resident serves such a consultative role under the supervision of a general medicine faculty member. The purpose of this rotation is to provide experience in the medical problems encountered by patients cared for by other specialists. This rotation traditionally focuses on hospitalized patients with major exposure to pre- and postoperative care. However, surgeons are increasingly providing care outside the hospital setting. Therefore, internists should perform preoperative evaluation and some postoperative care in the ambulatory setting. To provide a balanced experience in general medical consultation, this rotation should provide consultation in continuity from preoperative to postoperative care. Thus, the consulting resident should be available to evaluate the preoperative patient in the ambulatory setting and to assist in the management of the same patient after discharge.

Although the block rotation has been the traditional venue for general medical consultation, there are other ways to organize this experience. For example, a resident's continuity practice could be the venue for residents to evaluate surgical patients preoperatively. Postoperatively, the continuity clinic and its outpatient health care team could mobilize to provide postoperative medical care, and the resident could then provide long-term continuity care for the patient. Thus, the medical consultation role should include not only the inpatient service but also pre-hospital through post-hospital care.

Ambulatory Block Rotations

There are several compelling reasons for program directors to use ambulatory block rotations in general internal medicine as a central feature of the curriculum. Several afternoons per week in a walk-in clinic provide many opportunities to evaluate undiagnosed patients with subacute or chronic illness. In these settings, housestaff are free of the distractions of inpatient duties and can concentrate on an intensive learning experience in which they acquire many of the competencies of the integrative disciplines. The general internal medicine ambulatory block rotation can also be a "base of operations" from which housestaff can go out to brief, focused experiences in subspecialty clinics, in nursing homes, or in home care. Finally, ambulatory block rotations provide an opportunity for an energetic house officer to see many patients that need a personal physician. By referring these patients to themselves, enterprising housestaff can build a large continuity clinic practice.

Block rotations in ambulatory care give trainees the opportunity to become proficient in areas spanning the broad spectrum of outpatient medicine. While general medicine continuity clinic is an essential part of the internal medicine residency, it offers limited exposure to many ambulatory disciplines, such as ophthalmology or otolaryngology, with which general internists must be familiar. In addition, subspecialists may be the best teachers for certain skills. A geriatrician may be better than a general internist at demonstrating the functional assessment of an elderly patient, and a rheumatologist may be the best teacher of the examination of the joints.

Block rotations in ambulatory care also provide time to present a curriculum of important general medicine topics, including informatics, clinical epidemiology, nutrition, prevention, ethics, and structured teaching of physical examination techniques: None of these can be learned in sufficient depth in a continuity practice. A block format may also enhance learning simply by freeing trainees from the distractions of caring for acutely ill inpatients and allowing them to concentrate fully on ambulatory issues. This focus can be difficult to achieve on traditional inpatient rotations, especially in institutions that perpetuate the view that inpatient duties are more important than outpatient practice.

The most desirable total number of months assigned to ambulatory block rotations depends on the context of the other rotations in the residency program and on the priority attached to teaching key ambulatory competencies (see Chapter 8). Just as housestaff learn the fundamental skills of caring for hospitalized patients during the first months of internship, so early exposure to ambulatory medicine may form attitudes that lead a resident to choose a generalist career. Program directors should consider providing at least one month of ambulatory block experience in the first year of training.

The core of the ambulatory block rotation should consist of meaningful clinical experiences in the outpatient setting. Since even outstanding didactic sessions cannot substitute for case-based learning, ambulatory blocks in the first year might include a sampling of outpatient clinics that can offer the opportunity to acquire the basic ambulatory competencies. Block rotations in later years should vary this experience by allowing trainees to choose a few clinical settings in which they wish to develop particular expertise, just as they are able to choose inpatient elective rotations.

There are many outpatient experiences from which to choose. Such areas as adolescent medicine or home care, which housestaff too seldom experience in their continuity practice experience, might be appropriate choices at almost any institution. The choice of other clinical settings depends on the types of patients seen in the continuity practice experience and on the clinical resources available at each program. For example, if a continuity practice population included few HIV-infected patients, ambulatory block rotations could include a required rotation in an immunodeficiency clinic at some point during the 3 years. Similarly, residents who have their continuity practice experience at a veterans' hospital would benefit from experience in a gynecologist's office or women's health clinic. The program director can tailor a resident's curriculum to the needs of the individual learner by keeping track of the types of patient seen by each trainee in continuity practice and addressing any gaps in experience by selecting appropriate rotations during ambulatory blocks. The grids in Chapters 5 and 6 and the methods presented in Chapter 8 can facilitate this process.

The resources necessary to ensure optimal learning in the ambulatory competencies are similar to those required in the continuity practice experience, where patient volume and variety are of paramount concern. Many of the subspecialty areas will be unfamiliar to trainees, and subspecialty attending physicians will need to provide more supervision and guidance than their counterparts in a general medicine clinic. However, the subspecialty faculty must also be prepared to allow trainees to interview and examine patients whenever possible since active participation is a more effective mode of learning than passive observation. In addition, attendings must be prepared to discuss a range of issues pertaining to each patient—for example, differential diagnosis, physical examination techniques, and cost-effective methods of diagnosis and treatment. Intensive involvement by subspecialty attending faculty is particularly important in ambulatory blocks because of the limited time trainees have to master the assigned competencies. In 2 weeks of ophthalmology, for instance, a trainee may only see a few cases of iritis, but he or she should still leave the rotation with an overview of the disease.

Subspecialty Experiences

Internal medicine training has traditionally emphasized knowledge in organ-based subspecialties such as cardiology and gastroenterology. To gain more experience in these areas, residents frequently elect or are assigned to rotations on medical subspecialty services.

As is evident from the list of competencies, medical subspecialty experiences are essential to internal medicine training. The de-emphasis of hospital care has shifted much of the diagnostic and therapeutic subspecialty care to the outpatient arena. Many common forms of cardiac, pulmonary, and digestive disease are now seldom seen in the hospital, and the inpatient service no longer provides the breadth of exposure to subspecialty medicine seen a generation ago. Extensive exposure is not likely to occur in a continuity practice experience, which does not have the concentration of uncommon diseases necessary for such training. To learn efficiently and gain well-rounded experience, residents will benefit from assignment to internal medicine subspecialty rotations.

Traditionally, subspecialty rotations have often been "mini-fellowships" of one month, during which the resident functions as a junior fellow on the inpatient service. Subspecialty rotations that focus on hospitalized patients no longer provide appropriate experience in the management of important diseases that seldom require hospital care. Therefore, each subspecialty rotation should focus on the important curricular objectives assigned to it by the program director. The grids in Chapter 6 serve this purpose. Residents will achieve many of these competencies in the outpatient arena. For example, during a pulmonary rotation, the resident may profit more from learning how to manage complicated outpatient asthma than from learning sophisticated ventilator management. Although each subspecialty rotation will vary, the objectives are the same: to expose the resident to patients with problems that may not be encountered in the inpatient and continuity venues and to provide the resident with a deeper understanding of selected diseases and conditions.

A less obvious but still important objective in subspecialty experiences is learning how to use consultants. By becoming more comfortable in key clinical areas, the well-trained internist can utilize consultants' expertise in a focused and more sophisticated way. In addition, residents learn consultation protocol from the perspective of the consultant. Important issues include coordination of care, follow-up responsibility, communication, and information sharing. These skills are all essential to learning patient management.

There are many ways to organize subspecialty rotations. A block rotation permits total immersion in a field and is ideally suited for an inpatient-oriented experience. A 4-week rotation offers a good opportunity to gain expertise in a subspecialty. Rotations usually occur in the second or third year of an internal medicine residency program. A longitudinal subspecialty experience may provide better learning than a block rotation by extending over weeks to months to develop skills in assessing the effects of diagnosis and treatment. Residents can assume greater responsibility for patients that they will see for extended follow-up care. Program directors can structure longitudinal rotations to combine several subspecialty disciplines, as is currently the practice in some primary care residencies. For example, longitudinal ambulatory experiences in rheumatology, endocrinology, and women's health are possible in a 3-month full-time rotation. A block rotation in general ambulatory medicine provides yet another opportunity for part-time experiences in subspecialty internal medicine clinics.

To ensure an adequate educational experience, the rotation must provide a sufficient number of patients with a variety of clinical problems. The resident must see patients who are representative of the subspecialty and who collectively provide adequate experience in the competencies of the subspecialty. Ideally, residents should evaluate and manage the types of patient that will assure an opportunity to acquire each competency that the program director assigns to the subspecialty. Faculty should not expect residents to evaluate or help manage patients simply for the convenience of the attending staff. Rotations should provide an appropriate environment and adequate resources for learning, including easy access to a divisional library that contains core subspecialty textbooks and journals.

Supervision is essential for both patient care and education. On outpatient rotations, the attending physician either sees no personal patients or has a reduced schedule to allow time to supervise and teach. Faculty should periodically observe the resident at the bedside or in the examining room to emphasize the importance of history taking and physical examination skills.

Curricular needs rather than service requirements should determine the educational objectives of subspecialty experiences. Therefore, attending physicians must strive to ensure that the residents acquire the competencies assigned to their subspecialty. The ebb and flow of medical practice will make it impossible to have patient encounters to match every competency goal. Therefore, the attending physician should make use of case studies, computer simulations, videotapes, and other educational materials to supplement the exposure to actual patients. While the mix of patient experience and other forms of learning will vary each month, the faculty must continually monitor residents' learning experience and place a very high priority on achieving complete coverage of assigned competencies.

Community-Based Practitioners' Offices

The educational rationale for providing residency training experience in the community practitioner's office is compelling. Most internal medicine practice occurs in community-based settings. According to a 1991 Macy Foundation study, approximately 91% of all contacts with a physician occur in individual doctors' offices, organized group practices, and hospital outpatient settings. Office-based practitioners now manage many acute illnesses and exacerbations of common chronic disease that were formerly diagnosed and treated exclusively in the inpatient setting. In short, critical management decisions for patients with many common diseases have become part of routine internal medicine outpatient practice. While these rationales for creating a rotation apply to any ambulatory setting, there are further compelling features of community-based practice. Community practitioners' offices are particularly well suited for learning the important concepts of prevention, office management, population-based health care, and teamwork, and the important role of the patient's environment in health and illness. The hospital-based medical clinic is not an equivalent venue—the patient population using medical clinics is different from that seen in the typical community-based practice office. Perhaps most compelling is the career-shaping opportunity to experience the life of the community physician, which is often quite different than that of the academic internist.

Depending upon the resources of the residency program and the availability of community-based faculty, the resident's experience in a community office setting could be either a block rotation or a longitudinal experience. This learning experience could take place in any of the 3 training years.

The most important resource needed to make this setting an ideal learning experience is a motivated teacher who is well grounded in the goals and objectives of the experience and who understands the curricular role of this venue. Many residency programs design a faculty development program especially for participating practitioners. The patient population should be representative of a mature, general medical practice. The trainee should have an examination room in which to see patients under the supervision of the practitioner.

As with the other types of rotations, practitioners should select patients that will help the resident meet the goals and objectives of the experience. The resident should keep a record of patients and their diagnoses as a means of tracking patients and monitoring progress toward acquiring the competencies of internal medicine. As in all other training venues, the resident should receive timely, specific feedback. Many programs have used targeted faculty development programs to help practitioners become more comfortable and skilled at giving feedback.

High-quality practitioners who use their patient care experiences to identify their own learning needs must model this professional behavior for the resident.

Sites for Chronic Care

Internists have played an increasing role in caring for patients in nursing homes, in chronic care facilities, and in the home. As the number of older people increases, the nursing home has become a common venue for general internal medicine practice. The home has also become an important site for care that used to occur in the hospital. With the help of visiting nurses and other health professionals, internists may now manage many illnesses in the patient's home setting.

Residents should have experience in these chronic care venues during their 3 years of training. The most important connection will be through the resident's continuity practice. Faculty should ensure that each resident's practice contains a few patients whose needs require the resident to coordinate home care and make home visits. The resident's continuity clinic panel should also include patients who need care in the nursing home.

A training program will benefit from formal affiliation with long-term care facilities and agencies. A member of the faculty might be the medical director of at least one nursing home, an arrangement that would facilitate a structured educational experience in the nursing home setting during a geriatrics rotation. Home health care agencies, visiting nursing associations, and hospices are among the important organizations that provide the teamwork necessary for home care. While the continuity clinic can provide practical experience in this teamwork, it may be useful for residents to spend some time working with these organizations and learning their perspective in chronic care settings.

Elective Rotations

Each house officer needs an opportunity to acquire subspecialty competencies, either through required subspecialty clinic assignments from an ambulatory block rotation, through inpatient subspecialty rotations, or by other means. Many house officers will seek still greater knowledge of a few subspecialties. Elective rotations are the principal means of satisfying this need.

Program directors and subspecialty faculty should be prepared to accommodate the diverse ends toward which housestaff wish to direct their elective time. Some housestaff will ask for the traditional 1-month subspecialty rotation. Housestaff who plan to practice in a rural setting in which there are no fellowship-trained subspecialists may seek an in-depth experience that will put them on the road to becoming the "local expert" in an organ-based subspecialty. They may wish to have 3 to 6 months in one subspecialty, with experiences scattered over 3 years of training.

CHAPTER 8

DIDACTIC PROGRAMS

Purposeful Instruction Outside of the Patient Care Environment

The lists of clinical and integrative competencies that describe the finished internist will daunt even the most determined program director. He or she may wonder how to teach all this material in just 36 months. In Chapters 5 and 6, we describe how to assign the integrative and clinical competencies to learning venues and/or rotations. However, assigning a competency to a rotation does not guarantee that representative patients will appear and that residents will learn all they need to know. Even if residents master the clinical competencies, they must still acquire nonclinical competencies that have been underemphasized in the past and now must be considered core material. How will we teach these topics? The answer to this question rests to a large extent on a coordinated didactic program. The material presented in this chapter builds upon traditional internal medicine didactic programs, expands and enriches them, and makes them relevant for tomorrow's general internists.

Internal medicine didactic programs—defined here as purposeful teaching that is not directly related to specific experiences with a patient—have occurred largely in lectures and conferences. Lectures offered during the first part of the academic year typically cover emergency and intensive care unit issues and the most common inpatient problems that housestaff will encounter. As the year progresses, the focus on basic topics shifts to a similar series of talks related to common problems in each organ system and to common problems in outpatient care. These lectures occur at times that are convenient to all housestaff and are part of a departmental didactic program that includes other scheduled conferences, such as Morbidity and Mortality conference, Journal Club, Grand Rounds, and Residents' Report.

More recently, residency programs have begun to incorporate workshops and other active teaching methods into their didactic programs. These formats are effective for teaching many of the skills of internal medicine, including interviewing, physical diagnosis, counseling, and clinical decision making. They can stimulate residents' learning in medical ethics, humanism, and professionalism. These interactive learning experiences usually occur in smaller groups of learners and require more time than the noon hour. Accordingly, program directors incorporate these sessions into block rotations or arrange coverage for other duties so that many housestaff are free for extended periods of time. The challenge is to field a program of didactic instruction that covers all the high-priority competencies. With coordination and planning, program directors may find it possible to cover the most important subjects using the active learning methods that are often more effective than lectures.

In the discussion that follows, we first present the characteristics of several didactic teaching methods. Then, we offer suggestions for fitting the didactic portion of the curriculum into the rotation structure of a residency program. We should first note, however, the emphasis on didactic learning experience in this chapter does not mean that we recommend de-emphasizing rounds, morning report, and other forms of patient-based teaching. Experience with patients is internal medicine's most effective teaching tool. However, through the opportunities they provide for reflection, didactic programs enhance and expand on these patient-focused experiences. Moreover, they provide what patient encounters may not: exposure to and exploration of the full range of competencies in internal medicine.

Methods for Didactic Teaching

The most effective didactic programs use several pedagogic methods, including lectures, small group discussions, case-based teaching (for example, computer-assisted instruction, role playing, and video), and self-directed study with a mentor. Workshops are not a specific method but a format for other teaching techniques. We present a foundation to help program directors select and utilize the most effective methods. Faculty interested in learning more about these methods will want to delve into the literature of adult education and learner-centered learning.

Lectures

Long considered the standard method of teaching, the lecture has fallen out of favor among educators, who have become enamored of more active learning techniques. Lecturing, however, remains the appropriate choice for presenting a large amount of material in a relatively brief period; when the learner will use the material in the format in which the lecturer presents it (that is, it does not require practice, internal processing, or individualized assimilation); when the information is not available in other learning media or is unlikely to be accessed by the learner on his own; when the circumstances require a moderately large learning group; and when the speaker is an expert lecturer. Moreover, lectures can provide the necessary base of knowledge for more active learning techniques, which then provide an opportunity for individualized practice and problem solving.

Lectures probably should be no longer than 45 minutes. Short lectures that link to other forms of teaching may have advantages. Many of the disadvantages of lectures, such as the lack of learner involvement and failure to take into account the learners' base of knowledge, can be overcome by creative use of questions, visual aids, audience participation, and advance work by the lecturer.

Discussion

Discussion is a chief method of education for adults. Indeed, the facilitative style of teaching that is so vital for internal medicine depends upon it. Discussion is particularly suited for engaging learners in problem solving, encouraging reflective examination of their beliefs, and fostering attitudinal change. A successful discussion will review perspectives beyond those held by any of the participants; assist learners to identify and re-examine their own assumptions; and heighten learners' awareness of a topic's complexity and ambiguity. Discussion is the preferred method, therefore, for complicated or controversial issues (for example, those found in questions of ethics and values) and for topics that explore the learner's personally held attitudes and beliefs (for example, therapeutic approaches to depression or how to deal with difficult patients).

Discussion leaders often make the mistake of equating a discussion with simply facilitating a conversation into which they enter without an agenda and within which they refrain from expressing a point of view. In fact, discussions benefit when the leader plans the organizing questions and provides materials for participants to read in advance.

Self-Directed Study with Mentorship

Self-directed study is appropriate when individuals must learn a relatively large amount of easily accessible material. Learners can proceed at their own pace at a time of their choosing and focus their study on areas of need. Self-study is an obvious choice for bringing residents up to competence in areas of knowledge that they will encounter in a subspecialty office rotation. The responsible faculty member can assemble articles and book chapters for the resident to read at the beginning of rotation.

Experience suggests, however, that self-directed study is most effective when there is an effective mentoring relationship. Mentoring implies a richer experience than merely directing residents to an assigned list of references. As mentors, faculty attempt to motivate their residents to enhance their fund of knowledge; they promote a resident's development as a self-directed, lifelong learner. The most effective mentors both support and challenge; they assign tasks and set high expectations; they cajole and reassure; they praise and criticize.

Mentoring provides what is best and most rewarding about working with a resident, but it does take time. Every office practice is different; each seems to have its own rhythm and pace. Many office-based preceptors find that self-directed study with mentoring works best when they set aside time at the end of the day for in-depth discussion of patients and assigned readings.

Case Studies

The case study method uses prepared videotaped or abstracted cases that may complement residents' experience with actual patients. The medium can be the written word, videotape, or the computer. Case studies provide reliably what real life may not. It is especially appropriate when residents already have some knowledge but do not have the experience to see how to use that knowledge or to understand why their knowledge falls short of the requirements of medical practice.

The case study method requires a realistic simulation of an actual case. Cases should illustrate a clinical problem that provides a point of entry into a field of knowledge. The best cases provide exciting opportunities to test one's clinical judgment and diagnostic skills, while learning something important for patient care. The faculty should have these goals in mind when preparing a case. In addition, the learning venue in which the resident will use a case may determine how to present it (that is, incorporating the case into one-on-one instruction or exploring it in discussion groups). The case study method is effective in subspecialty rotations as a supplement to self-directed study and in block rotations where cases provide a rich method for initiating a discussion of the integrative and supportive disciplines. Many programs use videotaped cases to teach interviewing and other skills.

Adapting Didactic Instruction for Different Categories of Competencies

The Organ, System, and Population-Based Competencies
The guiding principle of this resource document is that program directors will alert the faculty responsible for each rotation to the particular competencies the residents are to acquire during the rotation so that the faculty can shape the residents' experiences accordingly. We expect that most program directors will assign a major portion of the subspecialty competencies to outpatient settings. Chapter 6 of this report contains grids that can facilitate making these assignments. Each subspecialty rotation director should receive a list of these assigned topics and then develop a didactic program to cover that material, taking special care to cover the competencies that may not be represented by actual patient encounters. Self-study with mentorship is likely to be the most frequently used didactic method as it is well suited for rotations with a small number of learners at a time. A formal didactic program will complement clinical experiences and should improve upon the less directive approach of encouraging residents to read about the patients they encounter and to attend conferences intended for fellows and faculty.

Non–Internal Medicine (Clinical Specialty) Competencies
A self-study, mentored didactic program during a rotation in these disciplines—for example, ophthalmology—is ideal but depends on cooperation from faculty in other departments. For the same reason, some programs may be unable to provide every resident with an experience in every primary care–related non–internal medicine specialty. Program directors may find themselves preparing the self-study materials with input from the specialist. Alternatively, a subspecialist can participate in a weekly or twice-weekly primary care lecture series. Yet another approach is to use lectures to complement self-study. A lecture series can reach the

entire resident group with material that brings everyone up to the same level of knowledge. Since most residents are poorly informed about these topics, introductory lectures make pedagogic sense.

Competencies Associated with Specific Sites

In rotations associated with such sites as ICU, emergency department, and medical consult rotations, residents usually work in teams, and the didactic program can profitably use discussion, case study, and other techniques suitable for small groups. Since different attending physicians lead these teams during each month's rotation, the faculty can divide up the responsibility for didactic teaching and sustain a fresh approach to their teaching responsibilities. In contrast, a subspecialty faculty member, who takes a resident into his or her practice several months a year, may lose enthusiasm if called upon to deliver the same series of talks or lead the same series of discussions month after month. An alternative to repeating a cycle of lectures is to videotape lectures and then replay them in a group that includes a faculty member who can stop the tape to make a comment or respond to questions (tutored videotape instruction).

Competencies of the Integrative Disciplines

Developing didactic programs for the integrative disciplines may pose the most difficult challenge for program directors, yet it is precisely for these topics that didactic programs have the greatest importance. The nonclinical integrative disciplines are likely to be unfamiliar to residents. Therefore, residents must acquire the knowledge, skills, and even the vocabulary associated with each topic before they can apply it to the care of a patient, which is the best way to fully assimilate the material. The grids in Chapter 5 enable program directors to flag the integrative competencies for which formal didactive teaching is required. Didactic programs provide knowledge that is essential for learning the integrative disciplines. The preferred format for teaching these subjects varies but is likely to include workshops that draw upon the methods of discussion and case-based teaching, such as video, role playing, and other forms of simulation. Two issues are critical for success in these didactic programs: The first is an expert faculty; the second is time.

The importance of the integrative disciplines more than justifies ambulatory block rotations in all 3 years of residency. These block rotations may include general internal medicine patient care experience, required subspecialty office rotations, and didactic programs that cover, among other topics, the integrative disciplines. Block rotations afford 1 or more half-days per week that can be devoted to small group teaching that involves all the residents assigned to the rotation. Most program directors, we believe, will want to develop a robust didactic program that covers approximately one third of the integrative disciplines in each postgraduate year, focusing particularly on the competencies that are not likely to be attained through clinical experiences.

CHAPTER 9

ORGANIZING THE CURRICULUM

This report is internal medicine's effort to anticipate the knowledge, skills, and attitudes that internists will need to practice in the new medical environment. At the same time, it is a tool to help program directors assess and improve their programs. The main purpose of the report is to facilitate the process of curriculum development in individual programs. A training program's curriculum is usually a product of a curriculum committee that includes residents, faculty, program director, and departmental chair. In this chapter, we suggest ways in which curriculum committees can use the competencies listed in this book to inform and to enhance their local curriculum development process.

A key to this endeavor is the allocation of training time, which is an inexact process. In an ideal world, program directors would know the exact number of patient encounters necessary to achieve a competency. From the frequency of such patient encounters and their insider's knowledge of the educational value of each venue, they could infer the amount of time a resident should spend in each rotation and each site. In the real world, however, these concepts are difficult to translate into practice. Patient encounters are unpredictable; the number of patient care experiences needed to achieve competency is unknown; and program directors must also take into account the need to cover patient care needs on inpatient services. Despite these vagaries, meeting educational objectives must be the organizing principle for curriculum planning for residency education. Program directors who follow the suggestions within this report will try to identify the high-priority competencies, assign these to preferred learning venues, and allocate resident training time proportionately to venues, based upon the number of high-priority competencies assigned to a given site. They will also develop didactic programs to address specific competencies, both integrative and clinical, that require non–patient-based learning experiences.

This process requires a series of operations. The end result may resemble one of the sample curricula shown below under "Illustrative Curricula," or it may be unique. The important point is that a curriculum should have an organizing principle. We have proposed the competencies of internal medicine as this organizing principle. No doubt some program directors will devise their own curricular organizing principles as they strive to change their curriculum to deal with the forces described in the introduction to this book.

Steps in Organizing the Curriculum

1. *Inpatient rotations.* For each year of training, program directors should first determine the number of months of general inpatient medicine, emergency medicine, and intensive care unit rotations needed to meet a program's service requirement, educational mission, and the accreditation requirements of the Residency Review Committee—Internal Medicine (RRC-IM). Program directors may wish to use the grid format of the competency lists to relate competencies to inpatient rotations. These relationships will give the program director a sense of the educational importance of each inpatient rotation and will inform the allocation of time to each rotation. For some programs, the linkage between outpatient and inpatient programs may affect the assignment of time. Inpatient rotations that include several weekly sessions in outpatient sites (common in several programs that have adopted the Firm System organization) will require more months.

2. *Population-based topics.* If the curriculum includes population-based topics (e.g., geriatrics, HIV), the program director will decide whether to cover these topics in specific rotations or integrate them into other rotations, such as ambulatory care block rotations. The Task Force recommends that program directors strongly consider covering geriatrics medicine in a separate rotation. Many programs may want to do the same for adolescent medicine, women's health, and management of HIV or substance abuse. Alternatively, program directors can create blocks in which two or even three of these topics share time with each other and with other clinical subjects. Program directors should determine the appropriate placement of these rotations in a 3-year curriculum and, based on the number of competencies assigned to these venues, decide upon the length of the rotation. We will describe how to integrate these topics into an ambulatory care block rotation.

3. *Community-based practice.* The Task Force recommends that program directors consider assigning time to community-based office practices, preferably ones that provide residents with experience in managed care. Time in a community practice can be a continuity experience on a block rotation.

4. *Teaching in ambulatory practices.* After distributing the specific rotations across each year of training, and accounting for night float systems and other logistic requirements, program directors should identify the number of weeks that remain in each year. The Task Force suggests that program directors consider filling these months with ambulatory teaching (rather than inpatient subspecialty teaching). These ambulatory experiences can include additional time in residents' continuity clinic, in ambulatory general internal medicine block rotations, and in subspecialty office practice rotations. The number of high-priority clinical competencies assigned to a venue will play a role in deciding the proportion of total ambulatory time assigned to each of these types of rotations.

5. *Electives.* The remaining time in the 36-month curriculum provides opportunities for electives. Residents who plan a career in general internal medicine may

spend the time on the topics that they have not yet mastered. Some residents, especially those headed for rural practice, may spend several months in a subspecialty "mini-fellowship" to gain extra experience that will prepare them to be the "local expert" when they complete their training and start practice. Residents who are bound for careers in subspecialty, hospital-based, or academic medicine may use their elective time to acquire more skill in the intensive care unit, in subspecialty rotations, or in research.

6. *Teaching the integrative disciplines.* The ambulatory blocks and subspecialty office practice rotations offer excellent opportunities to teach the integrative disciplines in seminars and workshops, as suggested in the description of didactic programs in Chapter 8. Program directors can assign the integrative disciplines to didactic programs within specific years of the training program, so that some are emphasized in year 1, year 2, and year 3. Alternatively, these programs can be offered to residents of all years as part of a 3-year cycle of learning experiences. The grid for each integrative discipline should facilitate the process of assigning responsibility to rotations and didactic programs.

7. *Primary care practice experience.* Continuity practice experience is both a core and a capstone in medical residencies. The program director will have to decide on the number of half-days per week in continuity practice for each year. To some extent, this decision should reflect the amount of competency-based learning that has been "assigned" to subspecialty clinics. However, the decision should also reflect the importance of acculturation into continuity practice and the learning that occurs when a resident assumes responsibility for patients over time. With these considerations in mind, program directors may wish to reassess the traditional model of one half-day of "clinic" per week.

Illustrative Curricula

(These curricula are presented as possible solutions to the challenge of organizing the competencies into a 36-month program. The solutions differ from each other, as do the resources, constraints, and missions of the hypothetical institutions. This resource document does not propose a single curriculum that will be correct for all internal medicine programs.)

Institution A

Institution A is an urban, university-affiliated, community teaching hospital with an organizational link to a multispecialty group practice. Its mission is to train general internists for primary care careers, although one third of its graduates continue to enter subspecialty fellowships. Its inpatient rotations are not linked to the residents' continuity practice. After following steps 1 through 7 above, its curriculum committee has proposed the following:

		Weeks
Year 1	Inpatient general medicine	20
	Emergency medicine	4
	Intensive care unit	4
	Coronary care unit	4
	Community (office) general medicine	4*
	Ambulatory block rotation	8†
	Adolescent medicine	2
	Outpatient psychiatry	2
		48‡
	Continuity practice	1 half-day/wk

* Introduces interns to off-campus practice of general internal medicine.

† Includes intern's own general medicine practice, 3 to 4 half-days per week; several sub-specialty practices; and a didactic program emphasizing several of the integrative disciplines.

‡ Allows time for vacation, night float, or other assignments.

		Weeks
Year 2	Inpatient general internal medicine	16
	Intensive care unit	4
	Emergency medicine	4
	Medical consultation	4
	Nursing home care/geriatrics	4
	Women's health	4*
	Ambulatory block	12†
		48
	Continuity practice	1 half-day/wk

* Outpatient rotation that includes office gynecology, breast cancer clinic and mammography, and time in a women's shelter.

† Includes extra time in residents' continuity practice (24 half-days); didactic sessions emphasizing the PGY-2 integrative disciplines (12 half-days); and 72 half-days of subspecialty office rotations, distributed according to the volume of competencies assigned through the grids for the following subspecialties: neurology, 16; musculoskeletal and sports medicine, 28; dermatology, 18; and nephrology, 10.

		Weeks
Year 3	Inpatient general medicine	8
	Emergency medicine	4
	Intensive care unit	4
	Coronary care unit	4
	Liaison psychiatry	2
	Ambulatory block	18*
	Electives	8†
		48
	Continuity practice	2 half-days/wk

* This ambulatory block emphasizes office-based practice of internal medicine sub-specialties. Accounting for extra time in the residents' continuity practice and weekly seminars and workshops, where assigned topics from the integrative disciplines are taught, 108 half-day sessions will be available for office subspecialty learning. Based on the volume of competencies "assigned" to each subspecialty, these 108 sessions will be distributed as follows: pulmonary, 16; cardiology, 22; oncology, 24; endocrinology, 16; gastroenterology, 24; allergy and immunology, 8; and hematology, 8. (Nephrology and rheumatology are taught in the ambulatory block of year 2.)

† Elective time would be used for individualizing training to fit each resident's career path. Residents heading for primary care practice could use this time for training in such non–internal medicine areas as ENT and ophthalmology; residents heading for rural practice could gain experience in such areas as pacemakers and stress testing; residents heading for subspecialty careers could use this time for additional inpatient or outpatient training.

Institution B

Institution B is an urban university hospital sharing a campus with a large medical school. Roughly one half of its graduates enter subspecialty fellowships, and one half become general internists. The Department of Medicine has reorganized its inpatient units into firms and has linked impatient and outpatient teaching by including 3 half-days of subspecialty practice each week (12 per month) during its inpatient general medicine rotation. Accordingly, more time is assigned to inpatient rotations and less to designated ambulatory blocks.

		Weeks
Year 1	Inpatient general medicine	24
	Intensive care unit	6
	Coronary care unit	6
	Geriatrics/nursing home	4
	Ambulatory block	8
		48
	Continuity practice	1 half-day/wk
Year 2	Inpatient general medicine	20
	Coronary care unit	4
	Emergency room	8
	Home care	4
	Subspecialty electives	8*
	Ambulatory block	4
		48
	Continuity practice	1 half-day/wk

* Residents choose two subspecialty consultation services during which 2 to 3 half-days per week are spent in outpatient settings.

	Weeks
Year 3 Inpatient general medicine	16
Intensive care unit	4
Coronary care unit	4
Emergency medicine	4
Medical consultation	4
Teaching resident	4*
Ambulatory block	8
	48
Continuity practice	1 half-day/wk

*During this month, senior residents work closely with, and help supervise, the third- and fourth-year students on the medicine service.

Institution C

Institution C is a community hospital located in a small city. It is affiliated with a medical school that is 30 miles away. It has a long tradition of teaching by voluntary staff and has begun to rotate residents into the offices of these "private" generalist faculty members for block and continuity experiences. More than three quarters of its residents enter general medicine careers, and many have remained in the local area. Institution C maintains both a teaching inpatient service and a separate non-teaching inpatient service. Residents in this program have begun to use a logbook system to record their clinical encounters. The program director uses this information to shape the residents' final year of training, as described below.

	Weeks
Year 1 Inpatient general medicine	16
Coronary care unit	4
Intensive care unit	6
Community practice	4
Geriatrics/nursing home	4
Emergency room	4
Ambulatory block	6*
Neurology	4
	48
Continuity practice	2 half-days/wk†

*This block emphasizes non–internal medicine subjects, including dermatology, gynecology, ophthalmology, otolaryngology, and psychiatry, with specific allocations of time based on the volume of competencies assigned to each specialty (i.e., competencies not likely to be learned in continuity clinic or in the community-based office rotations). Because of the relatively small size of the residency program, no more than two residents at a time are on the ambulatory block rotation. For that reason, the integrative disciplines are taught principally during weekly conferences and during special seminars throughout the year.

† One half-day per week occurs in the hospital-based clinic; the other in a community faculty office. Whenever possible, residents are assigned to the same "private" faculty member for their 1-month block rotation and for their second half-day of weekly continuity practice for their entire 3 years.

		Weeks
Year 2	Inpatient general medicine	12
	Intensive care unit	4
	Coronary care unit	4
	Emergency room	4
	Community practice	4
	Medical consults	4
	Psychiatry (inpatient/outpatient)	4
	Ambulatory block	12*
		48
	Continuity practice	2 half-days/wk

* This block emphasizes internal medicine subspecialties, distributed according to the method described for Institution A.

		Weeks
Year 3	Inpatient general medicine	12
	Intensive care unit	4
	Coronary care unit	4
	Emergency room	4
	Chief resident	4
	Medical consultation	4
	Geriatrics/nursing home	4
	Electives	12*
		48
	Continuity practice	2 half-days/wk

* Residents use this elective period to obtain training in the competency areas to which they have not yet been exposed. Residents maintain a log of patient encounters and, with guidance from the program director, use it to identify areas requiring further clinical experience.

CHAPTER 10

RECOMMENDATIONS AND SUMMARY

Future Trends and Their Implications

The education of internal medicine residents must inculcate a variety of new skills. For example, residency programs should now prepare general internists to anticipate the needs of a population of patients as well as to manage individual patients. General internists will need to become expert in clinical epidemiology; preventive medicine; patient education and counseling; and cost-effective, outcomes-based decision making. They must be able to provide first-line management of some of the diseases of medical specialties other than internal medicine.

Most of tomorrow's general internists will work in organizations and will therefore need management skills and the ability to work in teams. Medical ethics, legal medicine, medical informatics, and critical appraisal skills will become more important as the general internists' practice environment becomes more demanding. To practice medicine skillfully in an environment that rewards self-reliance and discourages use of the hospital, internists must have clinical skills at least equal to their predecessors. Residency education must continue to foster the intellectual discipline of clinical problem-solving. Residents must have a robust knowledge of human disease and experiences in caring for the most complex patients.

Medical knowledge will grow at an unprecedented rate in the professional lifetimes of physicians who are now entering practice. The general internist must constantly evaluate these advances to decide which of them will improve the care of the patient. Scientific literacy will be increasingly important, yet challenging to maintain. Equally challenging will be the increasing responsibility for managing diseases that fall outside the boundaries that once delimited internal medicine from other specialties. Expanded patient care roles and the prudent use of consultants will challenge the internist's responsibility to sustain lifelong learning. Residency training shapes the future internist's attitudes toward constant renewal of knowledge and skills, and program directors are reshaping their curricula accordingly.

The competencies discussed in this book are the skills that the profession believes are important for the general internist. These competencies are signposts for educators and residents to plot the 3-year journey of internal medicine residency. Signposts serve as guides; they are not commands nor should they be roadblocks. However, ignoring signposts risks loss of direction. The competencies described in this book should help the internal medicine community stay on course as it adapts to the changing conditions of practice by implementing new curricula.

With these new directions and challenges in mind, the Task Force offers the following recommendations.

Recommendations

1. A substantial proportion of residents will eventually practice general internal medicine. The residency curriculum should prepare them for this role. Achieving this goal will require educators to link curriculum more tightly to clinical practice than has been customary in the recent past.

2. To reflect current internal medicine practice, training should continue to shift from a predominant inpatient focus to include greater ambulatory care. More exposure to primary care practice (i.e., continuity practice) is one way to provide expanded experience in ambulatory medicine problems and in the challenges of office-based practice. Experience in managed care settings will be important. Subspecialty rotations that focus on the problems seen in office practice may offer a more relevant experience than inpatient subspecialty consultation rotations.

3. Residents should master areas that have heretofore received little emphasis in the curriculum, such as informatics, clinical epidemiology, population-based care, medical interviewing, case management, and team care. These and other integrative disciplines detailed in this resource document are essential for modern practice.

4. A variety of educational techniques and venues will be necessary to accomplish curricular goals. Didactic programs can teach what is not likely to be learned through inpatient and outpatient experiences. Didactic programs, often occurring within an ambulatory care block rotation, may be particularly useful to teach some of the integrative disciplines. Computer-based teaching methods can supplement didactic sessions and even simulate clinical situations. Subspecialty clinic rotations can provide exposure to types of patients that are seldom seen on the inpatient service or in primary care practice.

5. Local curriculum development initiatives should be deliberative and should involve departmental leadership, faculty, and trainees. The Task Force urges that this process be competency-based, not service-driven, and offers this book to facilitate what ultimately must be a local initiative.

Educational Initiatives to Complement the Curriculum

Education becomes a vital, dynamic process when educators invest in processes that bring curriculum to life. Outlined below are processes and relationships that, collectively, represent an opportunity for internal medicine.

1. *Relationship of the residency curriculum to the undergraduate medical curriculum.* Program directors should coordinate their internal medicine curricula with the curricular guidelines recently developed by the Clerkship Directors in Internal Medicine (CDIM). One way to cope with the increasing number of

competencies of internal medicine is to rely more heavily on learning in clinical clerkships. Program directors must be able to assume that residents have a solid mastery of basic data collection skills before they begin residency training.

2. *Faculty development.* Preparing faculty to teach new material, especially the integrative disciplines, will require considerable effort for many internal medicine faculty members. Faculty development programs are the key to maintaining high teaching standards and learning new pedagogic techniques as internal medicine moves into new curricular areas.

3. *Evaluating the educational process.* This report does not specify methods to evaluate a program's curriculum, but it does recommend that programs evaluate the impact of curricular change. The ultimate test of the internal medical curriculum is whether it achieves its goal of educating internists who are well-prepared for internal medicine practice. Measuring this outcome is essential, but it will take time. Meanwhile, the participants must evaluate a new curriculum as it evolves. Program directors and residents should develop methods for evaluating how well their curriculum achieves its stated goals. National workshops and demonstration projects are vehicles for dialogue between educators who are striving to make their curricula into constantly evolving instruments for change.

4. *The curriculum and subspecialty training.* A curriculum based on the information in this book will prepare residents for careers in general internal medicine. Residents who choose careers in subspecialty medicine or research will need a blend of generalist skills and other skills. New curricula must provide opportunities to blend general medicine and subspecialty training. As stated in Chapter 4, the Task Force believes that individual program directors will find the blend that is most appropriate to the constraints and opportunities of their settings. In this report, the Task Force has rejected the role of a curriculum arbiter that would specify one curriculum for all of internal medicine. This philosophy applies equally to specifying the content of curricula for residents headed for careers in the medical subspecialties. *Each program should design a curriculum that responds to the constraints and opportunities of its setting and the aspirations of its constituency.*

Implementing an Internal Medicine Curriculum

The implementation of a curriculum that takes its origins from this resource document will be challenging because the document proposes accelerating a process of change that has already begun. The inpatient orientation and structure of residency training has changed little since it was founded by William Osler. Hospitals and faculty have come to depend on the effective and inexpensive hospital service provided by medical residents. Federal reimbursement for residency education reflects hospital service rather than the pursuit of modern educational objectives. The process of implementing curricular change has logistic implications that faculty and hospitals will come to understand in practical terms. For example, the costs of trading inpatient coverage for increased ambulatory education are as yet undefined. Curricular change will require the internal medicine community to be patient, persuasive, and committed.

Curriculum is a means to achieve educational ends, not an end unto itself. The impetus for curriculum change should be a compelling need to produce internists that are better prepared to meet the needs of today's practice environment. Each program will have to examine its mission, evaluate its constituency, and make the case, both internally and externally, for change or for maintaining the status quo.

Summary

Over the remainder of this decade, health care delivery will continue to change as large, vertically integrated health systems emerge and managed care becomes more prevalent. Internal medicine practice will increasingly emphasize prevention and cost-effective patient management, particularly in the outpatient setting. Although economic pressures will determine the pace and direction of change, the profession must anticipate these changes and proactively define the evolving roles of the general internist. The ultimate test of internal medicine's capacity for change is how it responds to the expectations of society as it re-frames the education of an internist.

This report provides a fresh look at internal medicine and the education of the internist in this era of rapid change in American health care. Taken as a whole, the competencies listed in this report constitute a detailed description of the internist of the future as drawn by the internists of today. Hundreds of internists, representing many perspectives—academia and community; private, institutional, and corporate practice; the newly minted internist and the mature practitioner; subspecialist and generalist—helped to draw the picture that emerges from this report. If this vision of the skills of the future internist is responsive to the needs of society, internal medicine will have taken an important step toward preserving its central role in American health care.

The next step for internal medicine is to change residency education so that it produces a graduate internist whose skills anticipate the requirements of our nation's rapidly evolving health care system. This book is a resource document to which program directors can turn as they adapt their curricula to meet society's needs. Its central contribution is a list of practice skills that a representative group of today's internists believes to be important for the future general internist to acquire. In addition, it describes one approach to using these competency lists to design a curriculum. We propose a method for assigning specific responsibilities to each rotation and a method that will help program directors to focus and define their didactic programs. Program directors who adopt this method will direct the faculty of each rotation to pay attention to the competencies that they should help the resident to acquire during the rotation. They will also have taken a systematic, organized approach to the content of their program's seminars, rounds, and conferences. The key assumption of this method is that residents will learn more during a rotation or in a seminar if the faculty know their role in educating the resident and strive to shape the learning experience accordingly.

We hope that the report of the FCIM Task Force is the first step in a dynamic process of curriculum revision. We have described a method for achieving curricular change, rather than proposing a curriculum that every internal medicine program must adopt. We hope that our report is the progenitor of many different curricula, each responsive to local needs and resources. As program directors develop competency-based curricula, they will solve the problems that they encounter. We expect that future editions of this book will describe other ways to implement curricula that begin with a definition of what the future general internist will do.